THE HISTORY OF AMERICAN NURSING

Edited by
Susan Reverby, Wellesley College

A GARLAND SERIES

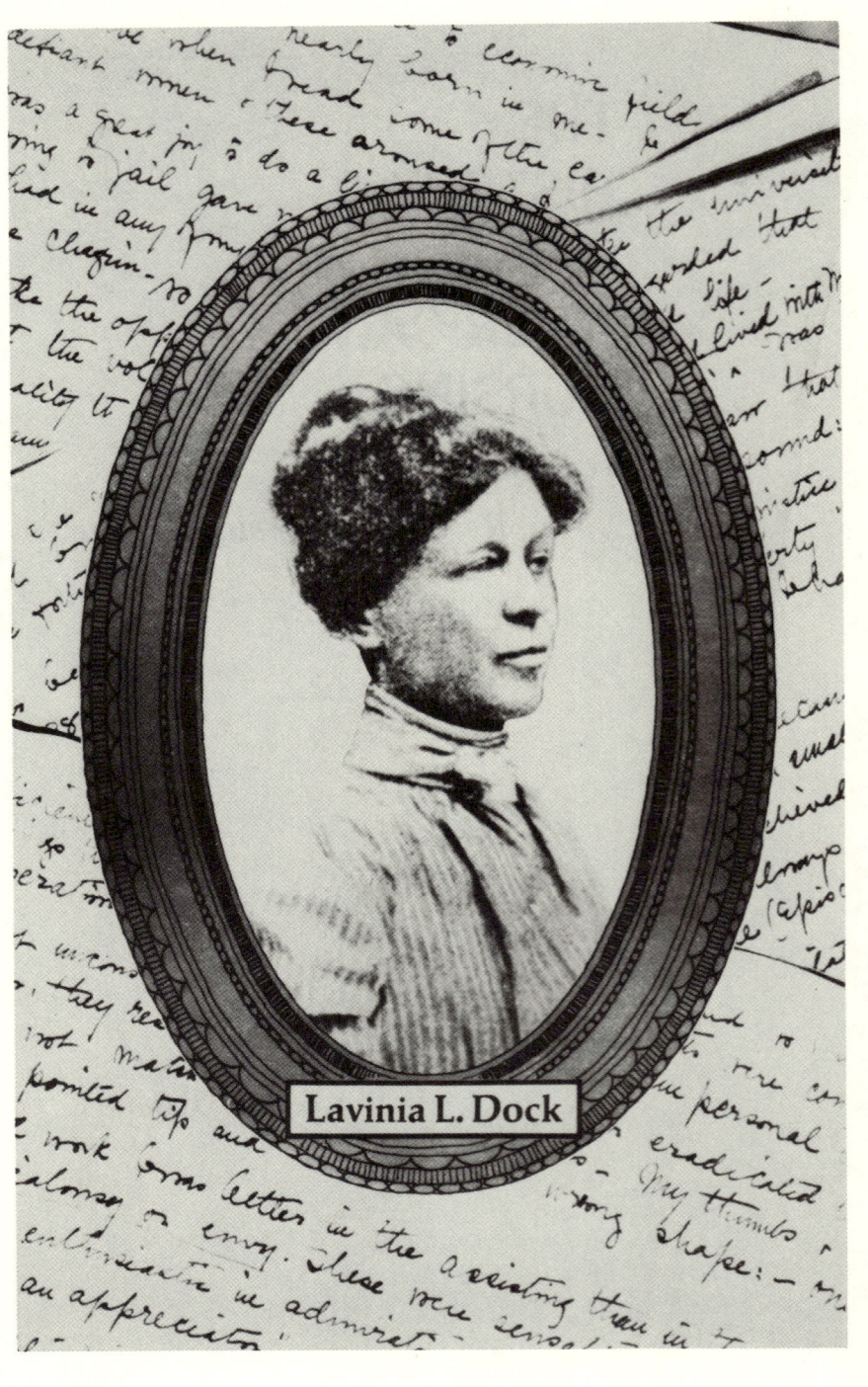

A LAVINIA DOCK READER

Edited with a biographical introduction by
Janet Wilson James

GARLAND PUBLISHING, INC.
NEW YORK • LONDON
1985

For a complete list of the titles in this series see the final pages of this volume.

"Lavinia L. Dock: Self-Portrait" is reproduced with permission from *Nursing Outlook,* vol. 25, no. 1, January 1977. Copyright © 1977, American Journal of Nursing Company.

The frontispiece is reproduced from the cover of that issue.

The facsimiles of *Short Papers on Nursing Subjects* and *Hygiene and Morality* were made from copies in the Library of Congress.

Copyright © 1985 by Janet Wilson James

Library of Congress Cataloging in Publication Data

Dock, Lavinia L., 1858-1956.
   A Lavinia Dock reader.

   (The History of American nursing)
   Bibliography: p.
   1. Dock, Lavinia L., 1858-1956—Addresses, essays, lectures. 2. Nursing—Addresses, essays, lectures.
I. James, Janet Wilson, 1918– . II. Title.
III. Series.
RT63.D63   1985   362.1   83-49183
ISBN 0-8240-6512-3 (alk. paper)

The volumes in this series are printed on acid-free, 250-year-life paper.

Printed in the United States of America

Contents

Biographical Introduction by Janet Wilson James

Lavinia Dock: Selections

What We May Expect from the Law (1900)

Short Papers on Nursing Subjects (1900)

Hospital Organization (1903)

An Experiment in Contagious Nursing (1903)

Some Urgent Social Claims (1907)

The London Meeting of the International Council and Congress of Nurses (1909)

Hygiene and Morality (1910)

Status of the Nurse in the Working World (1913)

Foreign Department, *American Journal of Nursing* (1916)

Foreign Department (1922)

Foreign Department (1923)

Letters to the Editor, *American Journal of Nursing* (1924)

Lavinia L. Dock: Self-Portrait (1932)

Lavinia Dock: Selected Bibliography

BIOGRAPHICAL INTRODUCTION*

Lavinia Lloyd Dock was known in her lifetime as a leader in the organization of the nursing profession, a settlement house worker, a historian of nursing, and a suffragist. She was born on February 26, 1858, in Harrisburg, Pennsylvania, the second daughter and second of the six children of Gilliard and Lavinia Lloyd (Bombaugh) Dock. Both families traced their descent from eighteenth-century Pennsylvania Germans. The parents inherited property in land, from which their five daughters in turn derived comfortable incomes until the great depression. Lavinia Dock, who remembered a happy-go-lucky childhood, had a conventional education at a girls' academy in Harrisburg. Both parents were liberal in their views: "Father had some whimsical masculine prejudices but Mother was broad on all subjects and very tolerant and charitable toward persons."

After her mother's death when Dock was eighteen, she helped her older sister in the care of the younger ones. She was, she later recalled, living "a very free and happy life" when she read

---

*Reprinted by permission of the publishers from NOTABLE AMERICAN WOMEN: THE MODERN PERIOD, Barbara Sicherman and Carol Hurd Green, editors, Cambridge, Mass.: The Belknap Press of Harvard University Press, Copyright (c) 1981 by Radcliffe College.

in _Century_ magazine an article describing the school for nurses at Bellevue Hospital in New York. In 1884 "Vinnie" went into training at Bellevue, the first American school to follow Florence Nightingale's principles. Dock survived the twelve-hour workday among the sick poor on the wards, learned all she could from the skimpy evening instruction, and graduated in 1886.

With no need to earn a living, she was free to explore. She worked as a visiting nurse among the poor, with the Woman's Mission of the New York City Mission and Tract Society, and then for a ladies' charitable society in Norwich, Connecticut. During the yellow fever epidemic in Jacksonville, Florida, in 1888, she ran a ward in a temporary hospital under the direction of Jane Delano, a Bellevue classmate. She rushed to the scene of the Johnstown, Pennsylvania, flood the next spring, and met Clara Barton. The real beginning of her career came later that year. While serving as night superintendent at Bellevue for six months, she compiled from medical texts the first nurses' manual of drugs. Her brother, George Dock, a medical school professor, gave helpful advice, and her father financed publication in 1890. _Materia Medica for Nurses_ remained the standard nursing school text for a generation.

In November 1890 she became assistant superintendent of nurses at the new Johns Hopkins Hospital in Baltimore under Isabel Hampton. The serenely forceful Hampton commanded Dock's loyalty at once. Dock took over the first-year classes and much of the ward teaching, making a reputation for her vigorous though fair distribution of praise and rebuke. Among the students was Adelaide Nutting, like Hampton and Dock in her early thirties. The three women were to become preeminent in the coming professionalization of nursing. Hampton was already advocating improvements in education and practice, and the establishment of professional organizations to control standards. At an international conference on hospitals, organized by the Johns Hopkins doctors in conjunction with the Chicago World's Fair of 1893, Hampton and Dock were featured speakers. Dock's address called for the separation of medical and nursing spheres of authority. As the meeting ended, Hampton organized the nurse administrators present into an American Society of Superintendents of Training Schools.

Dock stayed in Chicago to become superintendent of the Illinois Training School at the Cook County Hospital, the leading school in the midwest. In her brief two years there, she recognized her deficiencies as an administrator; she candidly recalled in old age that her "principles, aims, and endeavors were right and sound, but I showed no diplomatic skill in personal relations." From Chicago she returned home to Harrisburg, where, after her father's death, she spent a year in charge of the household so that her older sister, Mira Lloyd Dock, could take university training in horticulture. Late in 1896, Lavinia Dock took up residence at the Nurses' Settlement on the Lower East Side in New York City.

The community of women that Lillian Wald had created at 265 Henry Street was to be a congenial home for twenty years. "Dockie" became a member of Wald's inner circle. The affectionate mutual support of the Henry Street "family," and Wald's radiant confidence in their power to relieve not only human suffering but also the burdens of poverty, released creative energies. Dock's intellect came into focus with her ingrained humanitarian and libertarian sympathies. Caring for the sick among the immigrant poor was not a new experience, but the settlement nurses were virtually independent practitioners. With sick care went preventive care, health education, and pilot projects like school nursing that could point the way to public assumption of responsibility for society's welfare.

At Henry Street Dock rejected Social Darwinism for the philosophical anarchist Kropotkin's

theories of social evolution through mutual aid
and cooperation. She was introduced to the Social
Reform Club of trade unionists and middle-class
sympathizers, and met the eloquent Leonora O'Reilly.
The two women were soon organizing a women's local
of the United Garment Workers of America. Each
new experience fortified the feminism Dock had
absorbed by the time she was twelve from reading
"some of the earliest challenges thrown out by
defiant women."

The professional organization of nurses
remained her central concern. A faithful attender
and speaker at meetings, she was Isabel Hampton
Robb's chief aide in nurturing the Society of
Superintendents in the early years, and its secretary from 1896 to 1901. Her research into the
structure of other women's organizations and of the
American Medical Association laid the base in 1896
for a general membership group, the Nurses
Associated Alumnae, later the American Nurses
Association. When Robb and Adelaide Nutting, now
superintendent of the Johns Hopkins School, managed to establish a postgraduate course for nurses
at Teachers College, Columbia University, Dock was
one of the volunteer faculty.

Nurses knew her best, however, as a contributing editor of the <u>American Journal of Nursing</u>,
established by Sophia Palmer in 1900. A tireless

writer, she urged nurses to join together and stand on their own feet, while stressing their obligation to be socially useful. Most important, Lavinia Dock brought to the Journal an international outlook. A trip to London with Mira Dock in 1899 to attend meetings of the International Council of Women opened a transoceanic world of female amity and cooperation in the cause of public health. Dock joined Ethel Gordon Fenwick, the dynamic organizer of British nursing, in founding the International Council of Nurses (ICN), and was made its secretary.

She now became the communications center of the professional nursing world. In Europe she found the lines more sharply drawn between the professional movement in nursing and the medical and hospital establishments. Through the ICN she urged on the sisters in Europe in their challenge to medical authority, while in the American Journal of Nursing she conducted a monthly "Foreign Department," reporting the progress of nursing, public health, and social legislation overseas.

Of the elements of professionalism, nursing now lacked only its history. At Johns Hopkins, Dock and Nutting had taken note of the doctors' cultivation of the past. They planned A History of Nursing together, and the two volumes published in 1907 bore both names. The research, and the writing of all but two chapters, however, were Dock's. Pointing to historians' neglect of the "usual and homely," she traced the care of the sick from primitive humanity up through the ages. Women's autonomy, she found, had been lost when men took control of health care systems in the seventeenth century, bringing "general contempt" to the nurse and "misery" to the patient until Florence Nightingale came to the rescue. Thoroughly documented, the book conveyed the excitement of Dock's discoveries of women's past in libraries in France and Germany and the United States surgeon general's library in Washington. In 1912 she brought the History of Nursing up to date in two additional volumes by recording the experience of her own generation on four continents.

As she approached fifty, Lavinia Dock gave up nursing practice. Professional affairs still claimed some of her time; she helped Adah Thoms and other black nurses organize a national association. But nursing problems had come to seem only a part of the larger question of women's economic, sexual, and political bondage. An early member of the New York Women's Trade Union League, she walked the picket line in the shirtwaist strike of 1909. In 1913, in a major convention speech, she appealed to the American Nurses Association for understanding of the labor movement and a sense of sisterhood with other working women.

Nurses had taken many local initiatives in the Progressive era's campaign against tuberculosis, but Lavinia Dock was the profession's lone crusader against venereal disease. She allied herself with the physicians who in 1905 launched a voluntary organization to bring the forbidden subject into the open; she was one of the earliest members, only a handful of them women, of the American Society of Sanitary and Moral Prophylaxis. That year she began printing news of action against venereal disease in Europe in the <u>Journal</u>'s Foreign Department. Dock rejected "any treatment which would make it hygienically safe for men to continue a brutal misuse of women." Her real target was prostitution, and in 1910 she took a leading part in demonstrations against a state law which leaned toward regulation rather than suppression. In <u>Hygiene and Morality</u> (1911), "a manual for nurses and others," she called for abolition of the double standard of morality, for self-control by men, and for suffrage for women.

Lavinia Dock had been arrested for attempting to vote in 1896, but New York's police commissioner, Theodore Roosevelt, refused to put her in jail. The suffrage remedy was laid aside in the glow of hopes for economic reform, but in 1907 she enlisted in the Equality League of Self-Supporting Women, just

founded by Harriot Stanton Blatch with a program
adapted from the British movement.

Confident hope and the joy of battle carried
Dock through the turmoil of the next decade. She
ran a suffrage newsstand in front of the Equality
League's office and was "shoved about by police" as
a pioneer poll watcher. In December 1912 she was
one of the five women who made the thirteen-day
"suffrage hike" from New York to Albany, speaking to
crowds along the way. On trips to London for ICN
business she hawked suffrage papers in Piccadilly.
For the suffrage parade of 1913 she organized the
Lower East Side into a contingent carrying banners
in ten languages, and two years later was inter-
viewed while campaigning in a Bowery flophouse.
Dock's activities shifted to Washington when Alice
Paul began her militant campaign for a federal
suffrage amendment. She became a member of Paul's
advisory council, one of the few elders in this
group of predominantly young women. In January
1917 she led the first group of suffrage pickets
from the National Woman's Party headquarters to the
White House; she was jailed three times that year
and the next for taking part in militant demonstrations.

Few nurses or social reformers approved the
tactics of the National Woman's Party. Relations
grew strained; Dock moved out of Henry Street in

1915 and resigned from its board. When the suffrage victory came, the great expectations were already clouded by World War I. To Dock, war was the monster twin of poverty, spawned by men's greed and competitiveness; she determined that the conflict should have no advertising from the secretary of the ICN and refused to mention it in the Journal except to condemn it. In the early 1920s her Journal columns predicted worse slaughter, "perhaps [by] disease germs," if war were not outlawed. She shocked Journal readers for the last time in 1921, calling for the conservation of life through birth control, and praising Margaret Sanger "for teaching to poor working women what all well-to-do women may learn from reliable authority, if they wish it."

By 1922 Lavinia Dock had rejoined her sisters at home; the five women, none of whom had married, lived together in the country outside Fayetteville, Pennsylvania. She resigned as foreign editor of the Journal that year, and as secretary of the ICN the next. Dock's years in retirement were to outnumber those of her active career. Handicapped by increasing deafness, she seldom left home. Her arguments for the Equal Rights Amendment, introduced by the National Woman's Party in 1923, only widened the breach with former associates. The bonds of affection with Lillian Wald held, and she resumed correspondence with Adelaide Nutting, mending an old rift. Successive revisions, with Isabel Stewart, of an abridged History of Nursing grew burdensome, but the income from royalties saw her through the depression. She followed the course of the New Deal eagerly, especially in labor reform, hoping that what she saw was "socialism in the egg." The Second World War revived the anger of the First, and in the onset of the cold war she saw "conspiracy against Russia and socialism, everywhere."

At eighty-nine, Lavinia Dock was guest of honor, with Annie Goodrich, at the ICN convention held in 1947 at Atlantic City. Her tiny figure and her enthusiasm, humor, and resistance to eulogy captivated the delegates. In 1956, she broke a hip in a fall and died on April 17 in Chambersburg (Pa.) Hospital of bronchopneumonia. Through helping to frame the institutions of professional nursing, and by writing its history, she had done much to establish its identity. Her legacy was a feminist ideal of the nurse as independent practitioner and social reformer in a world free of barriers between nations.

[A very small group of Dock's papers is at the Library of Congress, which also has papers of Mira Lloyd Dock. A collection of family papers is also in the Pa. State Archives at Harrisburg. Dock's "Self-Portrait" of 1932, published in Nursing

Outlook, Jan. 1977, is the source of the autobiographical quotations. Her other writings include Short Papers on Nursing Subjects (1900) and, with others, History of American Red Cross Nursing (1922). Biographical details have been assembled from widely scattered sources, including Lillian Wald Papers, Columbia Univ. and N.Y. Public Library; Adelaide Nutting Papers, Teachers College, Columbia Univ.; Am. Jour. Nursing Coll., Nursing History Archives, Boston Univ. (including clippings by and about Dock from the British Jour. Nursing); Leonora O'Reilly Papers, Schlesinger Library, Radcliffe College; oral history interviews with Isabel M. Stewart, in the Oral History Coll., Columbia Univ., and with Alice Paul, in the Bancroft Library, Univ. of Calif. at Berkeley; Sidney Howard Bland, "Techniques of Persuasion: The National Woman's Party and Woman Suffrage, 1913-1919" (Ph.D. diss., George Washington Univ., 1972; James Frank Gardner, Jr., "Microbes and Morality: The Social Hygiene Crusade in New York City, 1892-1917" (Ph.D. diss., Indiana Univ., 1974); Allan M. Brandt, No Magic Bullet: A Social History of Venereal Disease in the United States Since 1880 (1984); Lillian D. Wald, The House on Henry Street (1915); R.L. Duffus, Lillian Wald (1938); Blanche W. Cook, "Female Support Networks and Political Activism: Lillian Wald, Crystal Eastman, Emma Goldman," Chrysalis, 1977; Ellen Condliffe Lagemann, A Generation of Women: Education in the Lives of Progressive Reformers (1979); Mary M. Roberts, American Nursing: History and Interpretation (1954), and "Lavinia Lloyd Dock--Nurse, Feminist, Internationalist," Am. Jour. Nursing, Feb. 1956; Margaret Breay and Ethel Gordon Fenwick, The History of the International Council of Nurses, 1899-1925 (1931); Mabel K. Staupers, No Time for Prejudice: A Story of the Integration of Negroes in Nursing in the United States (1961); Janet Wilson James, "Isabel Hampton and the Professionalization of Nursing in the 1890s," in Morris J. Vogel and

Charles E. Rosenberg, eds., The Therapeutic Revolution (1979); Am. Soc. of Superintendents of Training Schools, Proceedings, 1894–1900; files of Am. Jour. Nursing; Doris Daniels, "Building a Winning Coalition: The Suffrage Fight in New York State," N.Y. History, Jan. 1979; Ida H. Harper, ed., History of Woman Suffrage, vol. VI (1922); Harriot Stanton Blatch and Alma Lutz, Challenging Years (1940); Inez Haynes Irwin, The Story of the Woman's Party (1921); Doris Stevens, Jailed for Freedom (1920); Nancy F. Cott, "Feminist Politics in the 1920s: The National Woman's Party," Jour. Am. History, June 1984; obituaries in Am. Jour. Nursing, May 1956, and N.Y. Times, Apr. 18, 1956; death certificate from Pa. Dept. of Health.]

         Janet Wilson James

"What We May Expect from the Law"

Nurses who opened the first number of the American Journal of Nursing in October 1900 would immediately have recognized the author of the article on state registration. Lavinia Dock's materia medica text was already a fixture in training schools. But Dock's chief concern throughout the nineties had been the organizational base for a profession of nursing which the small group of training school superintendents led by Isabel Hampton was setting in place. As nurses felt their way in the expanding world of health care, Dock and her colleagues reached high for models, to the new women's colleges and to the medical profession, then just beginning its rise to today's high status.

Crucial, in Dock's view, were questions of authority, autonomy, and power. In a major address before the hospitals conference at the Chicago World's Fair of 1893 she had called for placing authority over student nurses in the hands of the training school superintendent. (See Hospitals, Dispensaries and Nursing in this series.) Later, in the pages of the Trained Nurse and Hospital Review, she had pushed the graduate nurses toward autonomy by denouncing directories (employment offices) and pension funds run by the medical establishment. Her research report of 1896 (see American Society of Superintendents, Annual Conventions, in this series) supplied guidelines for founding a general membership organization, the Nurses' Associated Alumnae, predecessor of the American Nurses Association.

In the essay that follows, commenting on the law for which New York state nurses were campaigning, Dock warned that Rome was not built in a day and correctly forecast the long succession of nurse practice acts that would be needed, adding to the qualifications and authority of the registered nurse.

WHAT WE MAY EXPECT FROM THE LAW

By LAVINIA L. DOCK

" Our human laws are but the copies more or less imperfect of the eternal laws, so far as we can read them, and either succeed and promote our welfare or fail and bring confusion and disaster according as the legislator's insight has detected the true principles or has been dictated by ignorance and selfishness."—FROUDE.

" Law as it actually exists in modern society is the aggregate of a system of rules by which a political community regulates or professes to regulate the conduct and the rights and powers of its members and its own interference with their freedom, and any rule answering this description is, if authoritatively promulgated, a law."—CENTURY DICTIONARY.

MANY of us have an indistinct impression that the " law" is something of the nature of a finished product, of which certain ready-made quantities may be procured as one orders household goods. One often hears the words, " There ought to be a law to compel" thus and so, or, " Such a thing ought to be forbidden by law." It is the natural attitude of the mind towards something unfamiliar. Let us realize that laws are public agreements which people just like us make and which we can also make. To have laws passed regulating our profession is only to do on a large scale what we now do in a small way in our voluntary constitutions and by-laws. We must first decide what we want to do, then find out what others who are of different opinions want, and finally by mutual agreement decide on concessions which we can get a good working majority to support. Even as to compulsory power, which is the essential characteristic of law, the difference is only one of degree: our voluntary constitutions have the germ of the compulsory idea, the difference being that this compulsion cannot reach outside of the association, whereas in State law the compulsion reaches throughout the State.

To be effective, a compulsory law must not only provide the penalty for disobedience, but must make provision for enforcing this penalty and for defraying costs.

Many laws, especially such as are meant to regulate the conditions of labor of, let us say, women and children, fail entirely to effect the desired changes because they have been so constructed that the method of enforcing the penalty has been left out. This point needs emphasis; so many people imagine that law is like an automatically working machine; that once passed it will keep on going of its own accord, protecting the good and restraining the bad. On the contrary, unless some one is enough interested to be responsible for seeing that it is obeyed, it will stand on the books forever as harmlessly as a verse from " Mother

Goose." "If the mere passage of restraining acts were sufficient to keep men from crime, or even in any great measure to limit it, there would be no such thing as theft, for there are enough laws against it." * Who then is responsible for seeing that law is obeyed? Whoever is injuriously affected by its being disobeyed must see to it. If the State is injured, the State will see to it. But if we make laws for our benefit, the State will not concern itself further than by providing courts of justice. Thus we find that in the best medical laws, the county medical societies are designated as being the bodies who 'shall bring prosecution for violations of law, and the expenses they incur are to be repaid from the fines.

We, if we wish to secure laws, will have to do the same. The only alternative would be to allow some other body of persons to take this trouble off our hands, in return for which service we would place ourselves under their control. This would be slavery, of which not even the shadow can be tolerated.

So it comes down to this: not, What can we expect from the law? but, What can we expect from ourselves and from the people all about us? They will not willingly allow us an advantage which they think will disadvantage themselves, and we may not disregard their interests in considering our own, but should rather seek to safeguard both, and so go amicably on together.

What, then, do we want to do? To establish a recognized standard of professional education. There will be a disappointment here to many, for we cannot establish by law our *highest* professional standards, only the medium,—only the fair general average, at any rate, at first. The secretary of the University of the State of New York writes: "It would be wise, in a movement for licensing trained nurses, to establish a State society and then to determine *minimum* qualifications to be exacted in preliminary and professional training. The object of the law will be defeated if the requirements are fixed too high at first."

Restrictive legislation affecting the professions, then, is not to be gained once and forever; this is another point for us to remember. It does not mean just one effort, but continuous efforts for the rest of time.

The American Medical Association has been working at legislation for fifty years, and the secretary writes: "The laws are *gradually becoming more stringent* [italics are ours] in the States which have adopted medical laws." Our highest present standards are the result of special intelligence and special advantages; all have not the same, and

* Proceedings Sixteenth Annual Convention National Association Dental Faculties.

it would be no more reasonable to expect all to suddenly conform to the highest, than it would be to expect the bread to bake without being long enough in the oven. We must first have the higher education, and then the law to protect it. The secretary of a certain national association writes: "We have secured laws in several States; . . . while these are not such as we would like to have them, yet they are an entering wedge; . . . the one thing that is needed first is good technical education before we can expect good legislation." And another: "It is worse than folly to hope to make men ethical by the law, just as it is supreme inanity to expect legislation to make them intelligent or learned; . . . we urge the abandonment of professional strife, the burying of personal differences, and the union of all in one common purpose to raise our professional standards as fast as, and no faster than, they can be firmly maintained." *

We have, as nurses, a fair average standard of two-years' general training, sanctioned by public consent during thirty years. We are developing a three-years' general training through the individual initiative and mutual agreement of those who have grown to this stage of progress

We may safely trust this element to go on distributing the leaven. It is instinct with the spirit of growth and needs only to be let alone. But we can *not* trust those who, from mistaken motives or from imperfect intelligence, attack our two-years' minimum. These are they against whom we must defend ourselves by laws which will forbid them to chip away a bit here and a bit there, like thieves at a cellar-wall.

Such encroachment on fair standards as a *six-weeks' theoretical course* in nursing, concluded by the giving of a diploma, which is now in existence in one of our large cities (not conducted, one is glad to say, by nurses), could be put an end to by a State association of nurses by passing a simple law requiring a stated time-limit, just as similar medical swindles, bogus colleges, and the like have been put an end to by the State medical societies.

Another sorely needed protection, towards which the "time-limit" of study, which is considered essential by all the professions, would not help us, is against the multiplication of training-schools in specialty hospitals and those of limited clinical material. To obviate this it would be necessary to specify in the law the variety of subjects in which a nurse applying for State registration would be required to pass examination. This is done in the best medical laws, but we would hardly secure such provision at law for some time to come, as it would naturally meet with great opposition at first.

* Proceedings Sixteenth Annual Convention National Association Dental Faculties.

The dental profession has successfully limited the numbers of dental colleges through its Association of Dental Faculties, and so maintains their standards: needless, however, to point out the difference between their circumstances and ours. Hospitals not only ought not to be limited, but ought to be multiplied, of every kind, special as well as general, and the training-school is usually a part of the hospital, not a separate entity like a college. However, that it might be made more so than it is has been repeatedly urged by nurses who consider these things, for the past six years or more. A system of paid graduates for private hospitals, post-graduate courses in large specialty hospitals, and a rotation of pupils from some large central school for the small general and specialty hospitals has been urged by nurses at private duty and in hospital work, by the American Society of Superintendents, and by the English Matrons in Council in print and in public discussions over and over again. It is satisfactory to see that members of the medical profession are now adopting our views and advising hospital managers to work out the plan. " First the blade, then the ear, then the full corn in the ear."

The secretary of the University of the State of New York writes, again: " It would probably be impossible to effect direct legislation to prevent training-schools from being established in small or specialty hospitals, from the innate American desire for personal liberty, and legislators hesitate to enact•such laws. The indirect method would doubtless receive wider support."

As to how legislation would affect nurses already practising, a study of the medical laws of the different States shows that reputable practitioners already established were in no case taken by surprise to their disadvantage, but were treated with extreme consideration. In some States they were not required to pass the newly established examinations, but received the State certificate for registration simply on the strength of their diplomas or from five to ten years' practice. Other States gave two or three years' time in which they might prepare for examination. The newly made laws usually provided that such steps as extending the course or amplifying the subjects for examination should not take place immediately, but at a given date from two to five years after the passage of the law. This gave time for accommodation to take place, and worked no immediate hardship. Such questions as moving one's residence are easily arranged for on common-sense principles.

EXAMPLES OF MEDICAL LAWS, CONDENSED.

1.

No person allowed to practise without certificate of qualifications from an authorized board of medical examiners. State and County Societies elect examining boards, one for State and one in each county. Each of these boards may examine. Qualifications necessary for passing are left to their judgment; no specifications in law. All those already practising at time of passage of act to be entitled to certificate of medical examining board without passing examinations. Penalty misdemeanor; fine $25 to $100.

2.

Regents elected for life by Legislature. Appoint medical examining boards from nominations made by medical societies. Expenses of boards met by fees. Qualifications specified in law: Age, moral character, proofs of preliminary education, college or high school or equivalent, or regents' examinations; four years from date this preliminary work to be more exacting. Four-years' course in medical college of a certain grade; e.g., any one registered by regents as maintaining uniform standards. Evidence of five or more years' practice may be accepted as equivalent, such substitution to be recorded in license. Men from other States where State board has standards not lower may have their certificates endorsed by regents, with all rights. Penalty, $250 to $500 fine,—or imprisonment, or both.

3.

Law provides two forms of certificate,—one for those already practising and one for future applicants.

Short Papers on Nursing Subjects

In this collection of essays we find Dock again wrestling with problems of authority and self-government, but now with new perspectives derived from her work at the Henry Street Settlement and her first trip abroad in 1899. Her pilgrimage to Kaiserswerth gave her a sense of the long sweep of history, and she now wrote with a new eloquence. Observing the authoritarian organization in Germany, in which women were silent, and the divided and embattled profession in England, she began to understand the obstacles to self-determination not only for nurses but for all women.

Back in New York, Dock's almost idyllic picture of the life at Henry Street shows us a "family" of women living as a cooperative community for helping the less fortunate, virtually independent of medical authority. In this setting she worked toward a new definition of ethics, a philosophy of social obligation to all classes.

A true ethics, she thought, would also help nurses learn to be more self-reliant in the management of their affairs. Returning once more to the vexed question of securing employment, she urged nurses to band together in independent offices and free themselves from the typical directory run by training school boards or medical societies which appropriated the fees for their own uses. Secure in the possession of a private income, Dock seems to have had small sympathy for ordinary nurses who hesitated to break away from a system which, exploitative though it was, did supply the private duty jobs on which their livelihood depended.

SHORT PAPERS

ON

NURSING SUBJECTS

By L. L. DOCK

SHORT PAPERS ON NURSING SUBJECTS

—BY—

L. L. DOCK

New York, 1900
M. LOUISE LONGEWAY
Publisher

Copyrighted 1900
By L. L. DOCK.
All rights reserved

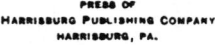
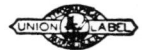

CONTENTS.

A Pilgrimage to Kaiserswerth, ... 5
Nursing Organizations in Germany and England,.. 10
The Nurses' Settlement in New York, ... 27
Ethics—or a Code of Ethics, ... 37

A PILGRIMAGE TO KAISERSWERTH.

The River Rhine lies broad and smiling before the little village of Kaiserswerth; its banks are low and rolling, and the evening sun shines on the great stone walls of the ruined Kaiserpfalz, which stands out majestically on the shore just at the turn of the road into the village street. Now is the time for a nurse of the modern day pattern to make pilgrimage to this remote quiet corner, where that system of work from which her own has descended was first begun by Pastor Fliedner in the early part of this century. Let her abjure haste, for on this side of the river there is no hurry; let her discard her modern strenuousness and relax the nervous tension to which she is used, and, taking a little steamboat at Düsseldorf, cut loose from the world.

Kaiserswerth is one of the quaintest of old-time North German villages. It has but two streets, one running at right angles into the other, and neither longer than three or four blocks of a modern town.

It has the prettiest little houses, their front faces scalloped and curving up into a point, white-painted, with every window filled with flowers. The streets are cobble-stoned and clean as floors.

The Gasthaus to which the traveller goes, is one of the prettiest of all, with low, timbered ceilings and a fascinating kitchen, hung and shining with brass and copper utensils of unfamiliar forms. The host, his wife, two daughters, and the little Dachshund, meet her at the door, as if she were an old family friend. Under the green arbor in the garden she will have supper, and, next day, all of her meals.

It is not necessary to tell again how Pastor Fliedner, inspired by the work of Mrs. Fry in the English prisons, and by an ardent, zealous genius for helpful work, determined to utilize the capacities of women about him, which were going to waste for lack of direction, and started what has since grown into the world-famed institution of Deaconesses, where the first modern training school for nurses was conducted by him with such remarkable system and thoroughness that Florence Nightingale, Agnes Jones and other pioneers of nursing in England went there for training, thus disseminating his principles throughout the hospital world of England and America.*

The new hospital at Kaiserswerth, the modern laundry, the handsome building occupied by insane patients, and other related establishments, all surrounded by the most beautiful and luxuriant grounds—more truly parks—lie at some distance from the village. Avenues of trees lead from one to another, and one might spend several days in visiting them all. But they are like other institutions, and one need not travel down the Rhine to see them. Rather will the affectionate interest of a pilgrim center on the old Mother House and its cluster of ancient associated buildings and gardens. It stands on the main street of the village. The oldest part can be recognized by its curved front, and the newer part, in old days the

---

* Pastor Fliedner had two wives, each greatly gifted with the special talents needed to bring the deaconess work to success. In the various accounts of Kaiserswerth, though the notable and faithful aid of these two women has been duly lauded, it has always been given second place, and it is probable that the first wife, Frederica, has never, until lately, had her rightful share of credit accorded her. It has been shown by an English nurse and writer of the present day that the initiative in this great regenerating movement came from the woman ; that her mind conceived the plan ; that her heart and courage prompted the first steps. (See " The Outlook," for Jan. 6, 1900—The Evolution of the Trained Nurse, by Mrs. Bedford Fenwick.)

hospital, is now almost entirely used by the young probationers and the oldest Sisters.

The Deaconess establishments, of which Kaiserwerth is the type and leader, undertake to care for their aged and infirm members. Naturally, the greatest number of the Kaiserwerth Deaconesses have families to whom they may return, but those without family ties come back, in sickness or in old age, to the home in the old Mother House, where they have pleasant rooms, beautiful gardens, and every care, and where they, apparently, have a peaceful and happy old age after their life-long toil. Here one may see these dear old ladies, all in the nursing uniform of soft, dark colored merino with a tiny light spot, dark blue linen apron, white collars, and gathered and frilled white dotted muslin caps. Some are sitting on the balconies shelling peas, and preparing vegetables for dinner; some are weeding the flower beds; others act as guides for the numerous visitors.

One is also taken into the rooms where the probationers are busy with house-work, mending, or study. They are kept separate from the general work of the establishment, and taught the principles and elements of their work by the older Sisters. Their own characteristics and talents are observed, and their fitness for special branches of work discovered. After a probationary period, varying with the ability of the individual, but usually lasting some months, they receive the general training during from three to five years. As, in our modern training schools, hardly a branch of work can be found which has not its root in this old school of Kaiserswerth, so, in this system of managing probationers, one recognizes the "preliminary course" so urgently demanded to-day by our teachers of nursing. One notices here, also, the origin of our "hospital etiquette," as the probationers courteously rise to greet the older Sister.

Out through the green and blossoming gardens one is led again, through the smaller garden where, in old times, "Mother" Fliedner was wont to sit or walk in the evening, her knitting in hand, and give counsel to the different ones who came to her—past the cheerful buildings where the old men live who have served the establishment and are now superannuated—through a corridor into the "Kaiserswerth Museum." Here are collected all the relics and curios which have been brought home by the Sisters from all corners of the globe, for Kaiserswerth, it must be remembered, has its Deaconesses at work in every part of the world.

Here is a huge stuffed crocodile, from the Nile; stone slabs, with Egyptian hieroglyphics and Assyrian pictures; models of Eastern temples, and of the branch Mother-Houses in distant lands; idols of every nation; costumes of every oriental style; thorns from the Mount of Calvary; curious natural products; the handiwork of barbaric women and things innumerable. On a long table in the middle of the Museum is a collection of articles picked up by the Deaconesses on many a field of battle. There are helmets, weapons, and accoutrements of war; knapsacks, cooking utensils, and flags. Finally, there is a case full of the medals which have been bestowed both on the Institution as a whole, and upon individual Sisters, for bravery in war and pestilence.

Away from the Museum and out across more gardens and a roadway, one comes to, perhaps, the most lovable and interesting part of all. Here, fairly buried in green, stands the tiny two-roomed house in which Pastor Fliedner began his work, and a little below, beside the old tower, is a row of small vine-covered cottages, in one of which Florence Nightingale lived during part of her stay at Kaiserswerth. Eagerly the pilgrim gazes at this spot, so full of interest and meaning in the light of all that has since happened. There are still some of the older Sisters living here who remember Florence Nightingale. "She was greatly distinguished," says the sweet-faced guide, "not only for her ability, but for her simple, unassuming ways."

Down the sunny road stands the little bookstore belonging to the Institution, where the photographs and leaflets may be bought that serve as memorials of the day. Reports of the work are to be had here, and accounts of the great Association of thirty or more separate Deaconess establishments, which have arisen through the example and after the pattern of Kaiserswerth. The delegates of the associated Mother Houses meet every year in Kaiserswerth, which they call the "Grandmother House." "We are firmly established under the control of the Church, and recognized by the State—nothing revolutionary!" says the dear old Sister as she offers her hand and bids the pilgrim a friendly good-bye. "Good-bye," and, without words, but full of many thoughts, the latter traverses the quiet street and goes back into the changing present.

NURSING ORGANIZATIONS IN GERMANY AND ENGLAND.

Although a short visit in other lands does not permit a traveler to learn the whole of the subjects in which she is interested, yet it usually inspires her with the desire to relate what she has seen, even though her tale be but an outline; and in the belief that nurses of the New World are interested in those of the Old, I venture to describe in a very sketchy way something of what I learned of nursing in Germany and England.

Germany comes first, both in my observations, and because it is from the German forms that the English and our own nursing systems have developed. I think this is a correct statement, for while it is true that the great English philanthropist and reformer, Elizabeth Fry, was the first to arouse that spirit of reform in hospital management and the care of the sick in institutions which finally culminated in the work of Florence Nightingale, yet the training of the latter at Kaiserswerth, and her establishment of the first training school at St. Thomas, which became to a certain extent the model for all others, gave the English schools, in modified forms, something of the organization and discipline of the great Fliedner.

It is most interesting to see, in full working order, a system as far removed as the poles from ours in the one principle of individual freedom, but like it in outer conformation, and containing all the germs of those changes which we have made. Then, too, there are to be found in Germany so many degrees, shading from their strictest orders down to organizations which are nearly free, that one can find there examples of nearly every stage passed through, in the development from the old religious orders of the Middle Ages to our modern profession of trained nursing. The very last stages of all are not found in Germany, nor yet even in England; I mean the organization and co-ordinated life of the graduate nurse, upon which we in our post-graduate associations and national union are now beginning to enter.

It is to be remembered that we nurses are descended in a straight line from the old conventual orders. In times not so very remote, no hospital nursing was done except by religious sisterhoods and brotherhoods. The hospitals were closely connected with the churches and were always built near them.

When Germany became Protestant, although ideas and beliefs were altered, forms were but slightly so, for forms simply represent custom, which we all know changes slowly.

So in Germany to-day may be found religious orders, Evangelical or Lutheran, which are almost as strict as the Roman Catholic sisterhoods. The obedience required is as absolute, the members or Deaconesses give up their whole life and enjoyment of personal property, and are not expected to marry. Others again, still religious and wearing the same conventional dress, are less rigid; the nurses are not bound for life but may leave and marry. Still the rules while in service are very strict, and the daily life could hardly be distinguished from that of the others. The Deaconesses never lay off their uniform, do not go to places of amusement, and have no choice as to their work, but go where they are sent and do what they are told. They work in hospitals, do district nursing, or are sent to private duty. Though there is always at their head a head sister or Oberin, yet the real control of these orders is in the hands of the clergy or "pastors."

On the street, whatever the uniform may be (often brown or gray, sometimes black), the Deaconesses may always be distinguished by the form of their white starched linen cap, or more properly hood, which comes down over the ears and ties under the chin. All nurses in Germany wear street uniforms, but the little hoods or bonnets of the lay nurses or "sisters," do not cover the ears.

As the Deaconesses grow old they are cared for by the Mother-House, and as they have no future to worry over, one usually sees on the faces of these women the sweet, serene, placid expression typical of conventual life. One finds, too, in talking with them that the problems of to-day, as we nurses feel them, are as totally unknown to them as life in another planet. All things are very clear and simple to them. People are divided into "good" and "bad;" those who will work and those who will not, and all that goes wrong is ascribed to Providence.

We can understand them, but they could not understand us. To them, our modes of life would seem quite lawless, even revolutionary.

Then there are in Germany next, in point of freedom, the organizations of lay nurses connected with large general hospitals. The finest and most noteworthy of this class are the Hamburg Nursing Sisters, at the great hospital in Eppendorf, and the Victoria House Sisters, in Berlin.

Of these two the Victoria House is the most "free" in this respect, that no religious test is made; whereas the Hamburg Sisters are required to be Lutherans, though exceptions may sometimes be made. As these two great schools are much alike in their organization, I will describe them together, and it will be seen that, though not under the control of the clergy, they are still close corporations, thoroughly organized for work and mutual benefit, but allowing little latitude for individual freedom, the control all being from above and the benefits compulsory. The Eppendorf nurses belong to the Nursing Association (Schwestern Verein) of the Hamburg State Hospitals. The objects of the association are stated to be: (a) To provide a school for training nurses, in order that the sick and wounded in peace and war may have skilled care; in time of peace the association undertakes the care of the hospitals of the State of Hamburg, primarily the New General Hospital, at Eppendorf. (b) To bind the graduates (Schwestern) together in a close union. To this association money was given by a wealthy citizen of Hamburg, to endow the "Erica" House or Nurse's Home.

The officers of the association comprise various physicians connected with the medical schools, an administrator of the fund donated toward the Nurse's Home, the director of the New General Hospital, and the Frau Oberin or superintendent of nurses, in an advisory or consulting capacity. At the end of her time of training the pupil receives the badge of the association, a red cross on a white ground, and signs an agreement to give not less than two years of service to the hospital. As a matter of fact, however, it is assumed that she will remain during her lifetime a member of the association, that is, subject to the control of its officers; and while this is not obligatory most of the nurses do so, as they are thus provided with work and otherwise cared for, whereas, to do otherwise, i. e., to go forth and work independently, means that they cease to belong to the association and thereby lose all its benefits.

The graduates or Sisters are now sent to the various institutions belonging to the State of Hamburg, and to certain hospitals and other institutions in the German colonies, in Jerusalem and elsewhere, all of which branches are supervised by the Frau Oberin, a woman of great ability and energy. These positions are not open to nurses who leave the association.

The Hamburg Association does not send nurses to private duty, so that question does not enter here, but in time of war or during epidemics the Association is prepared to supply nurses for work under the Red Cross, the Frau Oberin holding a prominent and responsible position among the officers of the Red Cross Society of Hamburg.

The Victoria House, in Berlin, is quite similar in its general plan. However, in the time of service to which the nurses bind themselves they may be sent to private duty among the rich or poor. This interesting school (founded by the Empress Frederick, and having a very beautiful nurse's home, with single bed rooms), has now a membership of two hundred and forty graduates, and nurses several of the city, university and private hospitals in Berlin; does private duty and district nursing, provides for certain colonies and undertakes to be ready for war and pestilence. In these two schools, then, we have the form of organization which, by simply dividing or specializing its functions and transferring a part of the control into other hands, is ready to develop into our system of training school and independent alumnae associations.

The State pays so much for the work of each sister employed in its hospitals; private institutions and private duty of course also pay, and from the income thus received the associations pay the allowances and salaries of the nurses (very small they seem to us, ranging from $75 to $125 yearly), and contribute to the old age pensions and sick funds. The arrangements concerning pensions will require a little explanation for American nurses to understand. Germany has a compulsory system of old age pensions and insurance for times of illness, which has been established by law within the last decade, and includes in its provisions nearly all wage-earners and recipients of small salaries, among whom are naturally nurses. The distinctive feature of this state law is, that the employee and the employer both contribute to the provision made for the future of the worker, the proportion of the payments made by the employer being in the ratio of about one to three, speaking roughly. The payments are very small, are made weekly, and are taken charge of by the Government, a careful scrutiny being maintained by government officials over the accounts of each individual. Thus one finds that domestic servants, as an example, all have their little books in which, so long as they have employment, the weekly payments are recorded by stamps. When they change positions or lose employment, the records are submitted to the proper authorities. Such nurses as the Deaconesses of religious orders, I was told, do not come under the state pension law, as their Mother-Houses undertake to care for them during life and give them a home. But others do, and one great advantage to the nurse belonging to a secular institution over independent life is, that these institutions, as the Hamburg and Berlin Associations which we are considering, take the whole charge of the pension arrangements for their members, and, by paying the premiums and adding to the contributions, are enabled to secure for their nurses better and more liberal arrangements than they could individually obtain. In the case of the Hamburg Sisters, the State, being the employer, pays the employer's share toward the pension fund, and the Nursing Association, acting for all of its members, pays the employee's share.

Then, further, these associations have elaborate provisions intended to meet the varying needs of nurses who may leave or become invalided before their time, as is quite necessary when these hard working women are kept in an entirely dependent position.

Is there, then, no further development to be found in Germany? Though I did not personally encounter them, I learned of organizations which advocate the entire freedom of the trained nurse after her hospital course is completed, and obtained the circulars and explanatory leaflets of one, established within a few years, which considers the subject more from an industrial standpoint than the older ones, and insists that the nurse shall choose her own employment and receive her own earnings. In such a system we would find the stage of development next before our own. The final step into organization of graduates as a means of raising the profession of nursing to a higher plane, and of educating nurses to a larger view of their duties and responsibilities, is yet to be taken. Even these movements for "free" or independent nurses are initiated by "pastors" of liberal views, and all text-books, lectures to nurses, histories of nursing, theories of nursing and rules of conduct for nurses, are written by men. An American is astonished at the silence among these women of the Old World. The superintendents of nurses in these vast establishments, women of immense ability and possessing authority in certain directions more extensive than any of our superintendents possess, have no associate life. They do not unite, write papers, or speak in public.

Still there is an undercurrent going on among women in Germany and among the nurses, of desire for greater freedom. Many graduates have separated themselves from the nursing associations and are to be found working at private duty in the large cities. Their lives are rather forlorn; the patients and doctors do not like them as well as the deaconesses, (or pretend they do not); they are meagerly paid and have not learned to strengthen one another. One longs to help them but does not know how. Their help must come from themselves and will be the result of a long, slow process.

Then there are the Red Cross associations, whose work is marvelously perfected in Germany.

I have often heard nurses at home say: "What does it mean to be a Red Cross nurse, and how can one join the Red Cross?" I will try to give some idea of what it means on the continent, and it will then be easy to compare our system in America.

Germany being a nation of warriors, understands what it seems peaceful nations do not always know, viz., that no government can do all that is needed for soldiers in time of war, but that the nation must help. So after the Geneva Conference patriotic societies were formed all over Germany, under the patronage of the Kaiserin, to carry out the provisions of the International Red Cross. They have various names, such as "Women's Aid Society," "Society of the Fatherland," etc., and are to be found in every large city and division of the Empire. They are all associated together in the most thorough way, so that wheels move within wheels with perfect smoothness. They have certain representation in a Central Committee, and at the head of all stands an official appointed by the Kaiser. They do not disband in times of peace, but remain thoroughly organized, make yearly reports of their finances, resources and general condition, and their outfits, appliances and general stores are subject to regular inspection by a royal inspector. Complete regulations are made for the various departments of aid needed for the army, and in time of war each society knows exactly where it has to go and what it has to do. Their army regulations are not, like ours, meant apparently to make it impossible to find out where authority lies, but there is a direct chain of authority and responsibility from the Kaiser down, one might say, to the floor-washer. The Red Cross societies build and maintain, in the different towns, civil hospitals where they receive the poor and where they train their nurses. The women who enter to train as Red Cross Sisters do so on the same general plan which I have described as being characteristic of Germany, viz., the modified sisterhood plan. They do not look forward to independent work, but give themselves over to the control and uses of the societies. They receive their living, clothing and small—very small—salaries. In time of war they are sent to the military hospitals, and in time of peace they are kept employed in the civil hospitals, or are sent out to private duty, the society receiving their earnings. When they get old they are tucked into some easy berth or live on their little pensions as best they may. They are not bound to remain with the Red Cross societies, but they are not eligible for war service if they leave. There is no staff of women nurses attached to the army in time of peace, but should a soldier be seriously ill and need skilled care, the military authorities simply send for a Red Cross nurse. The Government pays nothing for the services of these nurses. As the Secretary of the Central Committee said: "We exist to help the Government; not to have the Government help us." Many women living in their own homes and possessing means take a partial training in the Red Cross hospitals, that they may take a helpful part in time of need, and I have been told that in times of epidemics, when the trained "Sisters" are all needed for emergency work, these women have taken their places in the routine hospital work.

Of all American women and even, I might say, of all American men, Miss Clara Barton is the best known and most deeply respected in this Red Cross world of Germany. She went through this German training and through their Franco-Prussian war. She is familiar with their system, and they all follow her course as the head of the American Red Cross, and recognize her as one who has rendered great service to humanity.

It is now easy to see why one cannot readily become a "Red Cross Nurse" at home. We have no such system as this on the Continent, and thorough and admirable as it is, it would be both impossible and undesirable to introduce it in our country, for it is based upon an autocracy which we hope to leave behind. It would take from our nurses all that freedom which they have attained, and return them to the conditions of the Middle Ages. We can nurse our army either by a purely volunteer service, or by a paid skilled service based on voluntary agreement and contract, but not by women who are simply a part of the properties and the outfits of the relief associations.

The spring exhibitions which are given in the large cities by the Red Cross societies are said to be exceedingly interesting. They show models of all their outfits, hospital tents, stretchers, surgical, medical and housekeeping appliances, dressings, clothing, etc. I was not fortunate enough to see one of these, but in a small exhibition I saw a nurse's outfit, which American nurses may like to hear described. A printed list accompanied it, headed: "A Sister's Trunk with Complete Equipment for War Service," giving a list of the articles required, which were as follows:

Three chemises.
Three pairs of drawers.
Three night gowns.
Two flannel drawers.
Two flannel shirts.
Four pairs of black stockings.
Twelve handkerchiefs.
Two towels.
One hygienic corset.
One flannel skirt.
One cotton skirt.
Four white linen aprons.
Two gray linen aprons.
One rubber apron.
One rubber collar.
Two pairs of black gloves.
Two pairs of boots and shoes.
One pair of gaiters.
One pair overshoes.
One moiré skirt.
Two wash dresses.
One black dress.
One dressing sacque.
One money bag to wear about the neck.
One mantle with cape and collar.
Three fichus.
One sewing case containing thread, needles, bobbin, pins, safety-pins, scissors, buttons, thimble, tape, darning needles and cotton, hooks and eyes, patches for mending.
One writing pad.
One wine flask.
One note book.
Twenty-five postal cards.
One hand glass.
One toilet case, holding soap box, comb, brush, nail brush, tooth brush, with powder box, sponge and sponge bag, clothes brush.
One wash bag.
One round cushion of drilling to fill with bran or chopped straw (like a rubber ring).
One small pillow do.
One spirit lamp.
One lantern with candles and matches.
One case, holding glass, fork and knife, spoons, scissors, knife with cork-screw, twine, hammer and nails, thermometer, red and blue pencils, temperature charts.

One hat.
Two caps.
One coat.
One blanket.

One umbrella, made to fold up.
One knapsack with surgical outfit.

All these things, with the exception of the knapsack and the clothing worn, are to go into this very small steamer trunk, and every thing was there, down to the last pin!

That's the way they do things in Germany!

The knapsack contained a complete outfit for "First Aid," and is carried, if necessary, on the nurse's back.

From Germany let us cross to England and see how things are going there. Shall we find nursing conditions similar to those of Germany or to ours? Both, I think one may say; at least, the principles of both are there, while the forces which have kept German nurses in a state of submissive dependence and those which have from the outset placed ours in a state of comparative independence are in England openly at war. There may be seen in active controversy the old ideals and the new.

The dissensions of the English nursing world have reached us in America, but not many of us have paid sufficient attention to understand them. However, to say simply "Oh, the English nurses are not united; they are perpetually quarreling and are all divided up into factions" is not to get any useful light on the subject. It is better to inquire why they are divided. It is not really necessary to try to unravel all the side questions, minor issues, and subdivisions, for they are largely matters of different taste or personality and are in their nature transitory. But it is important for us, if there is a big question anywhere, a real principle, to get at it; for it must concern us as well.

Blocking things out, then, somewhat freely, it may be said that there are two parties in English nursing politics: those who share the views and aims of the Matrons' Council (whether they belong to it or not) and those who do not; or, to describe them in another way, there are those who uphold the principles and purposes of the National Pension Fund (whether they belong to it or not) and those who do not. Or, to describe things yet more clearly, the line of cleavage is between those who believe in the independence and self-government of the graduate nurse and those who do not. For the whole main issue in England seems to be on this question: "What shall be the future of the graduate nurse?" When the American nurses went to the Congress in June to take part in the nursing section, various excellent and lovely people were heard to say: "Ah, you are running after the wrong people. The nursing section is in the hands of a faction. The Matrons' Council is not representative." Of course, this sounds impressive; yet that word "representative" is a little bit vague. I want to ask: representative of what,—of conservatism? I am not sure that the Matrons' Council cares so much to be representative as to be progressive. I know that it does care to be progressive.

The trouble with this argument is that so few of the world's advances have been initiated by the "right people." It has always been the "wrong people" who have begun movements toward emancipation. The curious thing is that when they have accomplished their purpose and have turned their backs in death they are seen to be reformers. It always seemed to me it would be so much more sensible and satisfactory, and would also speak better for our penetration, if we could recognize the reformers before they were dead; and the thought does occur to me sometimes, when I hear the criticisms made upon this person and that person for what they are doing: "Why, that sounds remarkably like what was said of So-and-So and So-and-So," (thinking back over the list.) "Perhaps, now, here is a reformer."

Ultimately we will all decide for ourselves who the right people are in accordance with our own ethical and professional standards. If we sincerely and truly believe that it is best for nurses to be controlled all their lives long by an order or by the management of a training school, then we will believe those to be the right people who are working along this line. If, on the contrary, we believe that there is no more reason why nurses should be so bound and controlled than there is why medical men should remain under the direction of their colleges, but that rather they should receive the best possible teaching and then stand by one another in the best interests of their work, helping each other to work out the further problems of their wider world education, and learning to advance in innumerable directions of social usefulness,—then we will think those are the right people whose ideas we find congenial and stimulating.

In England one may take one's choice, for both are to be found there; and this is the disunity, this is the strife in English nursing affairs. The Matrons' Council believes in and advocates the things which American nurses believe in and advocate. It stands for the clearing of the ground around the matron or superintendent of nurses; that she should, in her own province, hold her own right and full share of authority; that the discipline and management of the nurses should be hers, not some man's prerogative,—and this, be it ever remembered, is the principle laid down by Florence Nightingale herself in her classical Notes on Hospital Management.

The Matron's Council stands for the abolition of private duty by under-graduates, of all wrong systems the one against which American superintendents have most set their faces and which is now in America fast disappearing. It stands, further, for the abolition of what may be termed the "sweating" of nurses, viz., that system which keeps graduates doing private duty in the control of the hospital, paying them wages and taking their earnings. Be it here, again, ever borne in mind that the mere financial aspect of this system is not its worst feature, but is, rather, of absolutely the least importance. The nurses are paid good wages and, like the German "sisters," they do not need to take thought for the morrow.

The real grievance, the real injury done these women in all kindness by good and loving friends and managers, is that they are prevented from developing; they are forbidden to have a life of their own; they are not allowed that sweetest of all pleasures, the pleasure of giving oneself voluntarily and freely to the work of one's choice. Their conscientious managers are like the old-fashioned father we have all met, whose daughters, tenderly cherished, never had a cent of spending money and had to ask permission every time they went to town. Then, as a natural result of this system, comes the Pension Fund.

The English Pension Fund is not at all like the German pension system. It has not the dignity of being a government affair, but is rather on the charitable basis. Those who founded it do not like to hear it called a charity, knowing that charity is an unpopular virtue. They claim that it is no more charity than an endowed university or public library. This reasoning, however, runs off the track; for an endowed university or library is not aimed at one class, but is meant for all people.

The Pension Fund assumes that nurses are poor things and must always remain so: that they do not know how to manage their money and never can learn. (A large part of the endowment fund, by the way, was given by an American man, probably in one of those bursts of international affection to which men seem prone.) The payments required of the nurses seem to us large and the returns little, if any, superior to the German pensions. I see no advantage in the Pension Fund arrangements over those of a good life insurance company or a savings bank and school bonds. The nurses who join the Pension Fund are immensely patronized by royalty (with the best intentions), invited to eat strawberries, and decorated with badges. The accounts of these functions in the Pension Fund organ make us squirm in our chairs; because these nurses are not thus honoured by reason of being faithful members of a hardworking sisterhood, but only because they have joined the Pension Fund. If it is, then, so advantageous for nurses to belong to the Pension Fund, why should they be rewarded for so doing? Is not, rather, the whole arrangement meant to blind them to the fact that they are being kept in subjection and their earnings taken from them?

Many English nurses realize this, and I learned of coöperative societies among nurses in London much on the plan of our nurses' club houses at home, where the members rent a house, pay their executive a salary, and hold their own earnings.

The Matrons' Council stands for the organization and self-government of the graduate nurse and for her ascent into varied positions of influence and dignity. It wants to see her on training school and hospital boards, helping to direct the education of future generations of nurses. It is not insular and exclusive. It has honorary members representing eight countries and follows with interest the nursing movements of all lands. It is cosmopolitan and believes in affiliating nurses with other progressive women who are busy with practical reforms. At home it has over one hundred full members, all matrons holding responsible positions. These things considered, the criticisms quoted above against the Matrons' Council seem to be of small account. Ideas outvalue size, and the principle of freedom is worth more than numbers.

It follows, then, as the conclusion of all this, that nurses in England are not organized into alumnae associations as ours are. Such unions seem to be quite unknown among them. They have the St. Barnabas Guild and some coöperative societies; but our republics in miniature, with officers elected by a general vote and a self-imposed government, they are not familiar with.* But the matrons are much interested in this development, for they know that a class of workers cannot long survive as incoherent atoms. Either they must be ruled by others or learn to rule themselves.

There is in England a class of nurses who take no part or side with either one or the other of the two main divisons of the nursing world: neutrals, going their own way, doing their work, holding with neither,—a steady-going and excellent set of women. Yet it seems to me it would be right for them to come out and declare themselves. More of them would be found on the progressive than on the conservative side, and why should they refuse the aid of their moral support to those ideas with which they are most in sympathy?

---

* Since these articles were written the League of Graduates of St. Bartholomew's Hospital has been formed most successfully on the lines of mutual development and self-government. St. Bartholomew's Hospital has always been liberal and progressive, and following its lead the nurses of England will certainly advance in co-ordinated life.

THE NURSES' SETTLEMENT IN NEW YORK.

Among the various "Settlements," so-called, in England and America, which are the outward expression of a unique modern discontent first embodied in the life and residence of Arnold Toynbee in the East of London, none is likely to be of more interest to nurses, especially to those who respond to other than purely professional notes, than the Nurses' Settlement in the great crowded tenement house region of New York.

Its very beginning was out of the ordinary course of events, for, whereas to-day people who enter "Settlement" life do so consciously, the two nurses who, fresh from their training in the New York Hospital went into the densely populated East Side to live in a tenement among the masses of foreign-born people, had never heard of Arnold Toynbee; they did not know of Hull House in Chicago nor of the College Settlement in their own city, both already established, responsive to the same urgent pressure; they had not even read "All Sorts and Conditions of Men" in which Besant and Rice's heroine lives among the most wretched of London poor, and "Marcella" had not yet been written. In a word, they had no idea that they were beginning a Settlement. Simply, of the two undertaking this new strange life the one who was leader had, in the course of hospital work, learned with horror of the conditions in which the very poor lived, and filled with the conviction that if such things existed she must be among them to see where help might be brought, she persuaded a classmate to go with her and try what living among them might do.

Friends interested, yet not a little perturbed, promised

to see them through, and they went to work in a systematic way by getting letters to the Board of Health and the various organized charities, in order to be prepared at all points for efficient practical action. In this preliminary work they encountered the College Settlement, where they lived for a short time, finally taking rooms in the fifth floor of a tenement house. Here they lived for two years a life fuller of color and incident than many a novel. Their tiny rooms were charming in the simplicity of clean bare floors, six cent white curtains and green growing plants. They did all their own work, except laundry and scrubbing, and got acquainted with their neighbors, their chief solicitude being to approach these less fortunate fellow mortals upon the neighborly and individual side, and to make their own impression as friendly souls before whom all the confidences and problems of living might be safely opened.

Their nursing was of course their "open sesame." Armed with badges from the Board of Health they explored the tenements, and wherever they found illness, offered their aid in the natural, friendly way in which the poor help each other. It did not take long for the tenements to become aware that there were neighbors of unusual gifts near by, skilled in the management of sickness, more than ordinarily hospitable, and competent to advise in all sorts of emergencies. No suspicion of being connected with any of the "Societies" did they allow, and gave no alms, though, in pinch of need, they spent money, or loaned it, freely, as the poor do with each other, to tide over a bad time, and always most generous were they with sympathetic interest.

"I came up because they said here were some ladies who would listen," said an old man who climbed the stairs to visit them.

Two years of this life went on, during which the attention of many people was drawn to what they were doing. Other nurses desired to join them, and opportunities of extending their influence were offered them by different friends.

A house was given them, of the old-fashioned homelike type still found on the East Side, situated on a quiet street once the abode of the Quakers, and not yet entirely given over to the tenements. Its substantial, three-story face has an open and serene expression, and in the rear, a pillared balcony overhangs the little city yard. Both without and within it is entirely charming. One would not say that every trace of institutionalism had been banished, because it never dreamed of getting anywhere near. Simplicity, comfort, and beauty characterize this interior, within which goes on a life so full, free, and untrammeled in its coöperative independence, that it is hard to know with what to compare it. Perhaps it is most like the pleasantest type of family life—a family, to be sure, composed only of women, each one absorbed in busy interests, but in no sense a community or institution. A little group of nurses first gathered round the two pioneers, and then a friend from the laity, altruistic and endowed with many talents, came to join them, and took a house on the same block directly facing it in the rear, so that the two little yards are thrown into one, and with another small plot belonging to a technical school this open space gives a garden and playground of fair dimensions, in which are swings, hammocks, sand-piles and horizontal bars for the children who, in summer, play there by the hundred, and also a vine covered arbor where the mothers of the neighborhood sit with their babes and drink tea or lemonade.

The two houses are used as one, and within the past

year a third house, accommodating a family of four, has been given to the Settlement, whose workers began to overflow its bounds. This new house is "uptown," in the midst of the Bohemian quarter, for the head of the Settlement believes in small scattered groups rather than in large communities of workers, as being better able to reach naturally and intimately those with whom they seek to become acquainted.

Let me try to outline the daily round in Henry Street. Breakfast is at half past seven, and unless guests are staying in the house, this is often the only meal at which the members of the family find themselves alone together. The postman comes: letters are opened and read, work and plans for the day are talked over and arranged. Afterwards the rooms are set in order; new cases that have come in are distributed by the head of the family, and the nurses go off on their rounds. The entire day is spent in caring for the sick; and in following out the different lines of work which develop from this, the primary one. The nursing is of course much like the work of district nurses in general, except for the entire absence of any kind of restrictive regulation. Each nurse manages her patients and arranges her time according to her best judgment, and all points of interest, knotty problems, and difficult situations are talked over and settled in family council. The calls usually come from the people themselves, though charitable agencies, clergymen, and physicians furnish a certain percentage. Often the nurse is sent for before a doctor is called, and then, if one is needed, she decides whether to apply at the Dispensary, or to submit the patient's case to one of the best uptown specialists, or to advise hospital care.

The patients being usually of a poverty which makes life a pitiful struggle even at the best, the nurses' care is freely given, with the exception of one who devotes her whole time to a service among those of more means, who would not ask for free nursing. This nurse's patients always pay for their nursing at the rate of twenty-five or thirty cents an hour. Beside the professional care of the invalid, all the circumstances of the family, so quickly learned in this intimate relation, become the nurse's interest, and, so far as is possible, her concern, and through the acquaintance thus established, she is sometimes able to open the door of a different life to one or another; to bring longed-for but hitherto unattainable opportunities within reach of different ones who had been by circumstances deprived of all for which nature had fitted them. As the Settlement family is quite a permanent one, its members entering for indefinite periods and never wishing to leave, the nurses form real friendships with their people, who call upon them in every emergency, year in and year out. In addition to her nursing, each one takes up some special work of her own according to her talent. What this may be will appear after luncheon to which we now return and where one usually finds some visitor or visitors interested and interesting, for no dull or stupid people ever appear at the Settlement. Those who come there have some work or purpose in life and feel a love for it in its various aspects.

In the afternoon, nursing work is finished, it may be in one or two hours, or not until dinner time, and the specialties are pursued. One nurse, skilled in the Yiddish dialect, teaches a class of foreign-born mothers in simple home nursing and hygiene. These are the poorest and most hard worked of women and who have had the scantiest portion of the world's advantages. They have come from Russia too late in life to learn English, and can only understand their own curious jargon. They come weekly to their class, and after the lesson is over the samovar is placed upon the table and they drink tea. Visitors come in sometimes to sing and play to them, and reminiscences of Russian songs and folk-lore are revived in their minds. This lasts all through the winter, and in the summer the social part is continued in the garden. Another class is of English-speaking mothers, conducted on the same lines, and after they have had the nursing course, a series of cooking lessons in the big old-fashioned kitchen of the second house, where they sit down to a cozy, clean table with the prettiest of cheap dishes for object lessons, and enjoy the simple, well-cooked food made from the least expensive materials, and designed to show them how for the same amount of money that they themselves might spend, they can prepare dishes more attractive and toothsome than those they usually have.

These mothers are also of the very poor, though with more hope and aspiration than those who speak no English. They dearly love their classes, and call themselves the G. T. C., the Good Times Club. To those who know how sorely stinted in good times their lives are, there is unconscious pathos in this title. These mothers pay five cents a week for their cooking lessons.

Another nurse has for several years conducted a club of girls of fourteen and fifteen, the youngest in the ranks of woman wage-earners, and has given them in turn lessons in house-work, simple rules of hygiene and care of the sick, cooking, and physical culture, besides being older sister and adviser to them all. Another course of nursing lessons which is paid for at the rate of five cents a lesson is given in the evenings to more advanced young women and mothers of superior intelligence.

The nurse who is head of the house is endowed with all the social genius that could be required in such a life, and it would be difficult to enumerate the various branches of her activity. She is the fortunate possessor of a touchstone which reveals to her the best and finest possibilities of the natures about her, often quite unsuspected by those of less discernment, and this, combined with that best of all practical talents—the gift for bringing people and opportunities, the work and the workers, together—has enabled her to set free a multitude of energies, many of which strike their roots within the hospitable walls of the Settlement. The "lay member" who has had an unusually wide and varied social experience of the best kind, throws open her house to every demand made upon it, and is constantly busy in organizing some fun or frolic for the young people—a Kinder symphony, theatricals, recitations, or a musical party. A kindergarten occupies one floor in the mornings, the teachers of which are supplied by the New York Kindergarten Association, and their functions are among the prettiest that take place in the house. They have "mothers' parties" once a month, when the mothers learn the children's games and the ideas that underlie them. The "alumnae" of the kindergarten also meet once a week—tots who have been promoted to the public school but still love their kindergarten ways. Lecturers find audiences there and many clubs, classes, and re-unions come to the Settlement, being conducted by outside people, among which are classes in kitchen-garden work for little girls, cooking and sewing classes for older ones, debating clubs, a Shakespeare class for young women, special pupils with their teachers, and, for a year's experiment, a little shirtshop where unskilled sewing girls were taught to be skilled and capable of making a complete garment. A reading and study room for boys and young men is also in this house, greatly frequented, and particularly dear to the hearts of the Settlement is a club of boys led by the head worker, who study the lives of American heroes, and, under the influence which guides them, possess an ethical standard which would shame many a respectable citizen.

The "uptown" house meantime leads a similar life, and this winter a large school building belonging to the Children's Aid Society has been opened in the evening, with reading and game rooms for older boys and men, under the direction of the Settlement. Amidst the nursing and regular work that goes on, the social life is one of rare privilege and charm. Not only are interesting people from uptown and elsewhere to be met in the Settlement, but all the currents of East Side life run through and across it. Most valued among the family friends are leaders in the world of labor—soldiers of the industrial army—both women and men, who come intimately to the house, and whose work and problems are household words. The poet of the sweat-shops, whose pathetic verses have lately been translated and edited by a professor at Harvard, lived near by, and has read his poems there while men of literary fame listened, impressed and moved; young Russian and Yiddish writers come there, and aspiring young musicians full of talent and enthusiasm.

The neighborhood abounds with young men and women of fine intellectual gifts, who combine the hard work of the wage-earner with the capacity of holding their own in deep debate and discussion—in a word, here one has the opportunity of learning at first hand the movements and tendencies of modern life from the people who are working them out. Questions of municipal management, the schools and educational problems, industrial and economic conditions, the various directions in which social reforms are trying to develop; all these are being lived by the people who come to the Settlement, and this daily contact with the real things that are going on in the world gives an indescribable charm and fascination to the life. One seems, here, to be at the very heart of things.

The practical side is sure to occur to nurses, and they will now ask "how is all this supported and kept going?" One naturally thinks of executive boards, of committees, reports, and all that sort of thing, but here there is absolutely nothing of the kind. The Settlement is entirely elastic and uncrystallized. It has never been hampered by any formula or code. There is no outside management, no committee of ladies, no board of directors. No public or formal reports are ever issued, no appeals are ever made for money. Even in the daily press the head of the house, with great skill and tact, avoids "writing up." Only in papers or magazines having some bond of interest does the Settlement go into print.

The houses are given, and provision for the nurse is made in the form of fellowships, offered by different persons who are interested and want to help. One is given by the Directors of the Presbyterian Hospital and the Nurses' Alumnae Association of the training school. Nurses frequently offer their services for a month or two, or come there and pay their board to get an insight into the work. Eleven people constitute the two regular families, and they share alike in the expenses of living, no fixed allowance or stated sum being attempted. One member undertakes the housekeeping, sees the people who come on all sorts of errands, and presides in the little dispensary where appliances of all kinds are kept on hand for emergencies, and where supplies of clothing and conveniences for the sick are stored, to be carried out and used or loaned by the nurses.

An "Emergency Fund" to meet the incidental expenses of district nursing and Settlement work is well remembered by sympathetic friends.

Last and best of the gifts made by generous friends to the Settlement has been a country house, also presided over by a nurse. Here, all the year round, winter as well as summer, guests are welcomed and entertained; the tired mothers, worn and pallid young girls, and children recovering from illness. No time limit is set for these visits, only the need of the visitor, and this opportunity is so enjoyed that "The Country House" is looked upon as one of the chief joys and satisfactions of the whole work.

ETHICS—OR A CODE OF ETHICS?

Some few years ago, I wrote an article addressed to nurses, in which, according to the best of my ability at that time, was advocated the framing of a Code of Ethics as one of the first duties of an organized association of nurses. I remember that at the time a liberal-minded man belonging to those who are by profession our superior officers warned me as follows: "The Code of Ethics of the medical profession has been the cause of quarrelling, unbrotherly feelings and contentions innumerable. Be good women but do not bother with a Code of Ethics."

I thought then only that he did not take us seriously enough. Now, however, I am obliged to ask myself "what, exactly, could a Code of Ethics be?" A Code of Ethics for the nursing profession. I withdraw the phrase. For what are ethics and can they be codified? Do we aim at ethical exclusiveness and shall our ethical development be bounded or limited by a code? "Code" suggests statutes, infringements, penalties, antagonisms. If we have the ethics, we will not need a code. The code is to regulate those who have no ethics, and in proportion as ethical principles are made a part of our natures and lives, our codes and restrictions will shrivel away and die the death of inanition. Shall we then have no rules and regulations? Are we supposed to imagine that we can at once cast off all restrictions and enter upon a millenium of perfect professional conduct? Not quite that—while regulations are really helpful in guiding any of our associates, let us have them, to prop up the steps of those who are young in self-government or feeble in self-control, but let us not call them ethics. Let us call them our mechanical working methods, labor-saving devices, temporary expedients, to be thrown away as soon as they become clumsy or old-fashioned; for if we call them ethics we may perhaps come to believe that they are all there is of ethics, and presently be worshipping the code rather than the thing,—so unreasoning a reverence is there in our souls for statutes, fines, and punishments; so exaggerated a notion of the potency of drafted laws; so strong a tendency to make rules the end and aim of life rather than simply conveniences, changeable contrivances.

Ethical life is more than maxims, just as intellectual life is more than book-learning. It is far more comprehensive than we now even dream, for in our work so far we have not paid much attention to it; possibly, for one reason because we have been supposing that we were to learn everything in the training schools, and afterwards be finished,—our education completed. But it is not rational to suppose that our training school teaching could be more than the preparation, the ground-work of our professional life. Our self-conducted associations are the true schools for our broader education. Here we may take up the study of ethics, sharpen our perceptions, and learn to form our judgments. Such study, if taken in a wide sense, will end only with our life-times, and will not be completed then.

Where shall one begin to study ethics?

We have had so much said to us, and written to us, didactically, under the head of ethics, which is not ethics at all. There is, for instance, etiquette. It must surely be acknowledged, that, overlooking small failings and considering our training schools as a whole, the practical spirit which pervades them of devotion to duty, and placing this duty before everything else, is of quite unsurpassable fineness and leaves no room for criticism, being unassuming, unselfish, and in fact unconscious of its own readiness to serve. Yet it is usually an inarticulate spirit, rarely expressing itself, and the audible theoretical teaching aside from the technicalities which one hears in the training school, is teaching in etiquette.

Let no one deride or belittle etiquette; it has its place, a very important one. However it is not to be mistaken for ethics.

Etiquette, used, needless to say, within reasonable bounds, is like a common language. Its purpose is to avoid confusion in daily life and to introduce order by establishing one definite and generally understood set of good manners in the place of two or three hundred kinds of good manners, which, like different languages, may only be understood by those who use them. The nurse who sits rocking in her chair when the doctor enters may feel just as courteous in her heart as the one who rises, but the doctor will understand the one, and will not understand the other.

Many other working details which we have been wont to regard perhaps too seriously as indicative of ethics are not such at all, but simply matters of taste; for instance, the subject of dress. Here is a nurse who never wears a uniform. Here is one who always wears it within doors, and there is still another who always wears it on the street as well. Much disagreement of opinion there may be involved, but no question of ethics. The one in uniform may look better, but dare she conclude that hers is a condition of ethical superiority? Let us recognize etiquette, and acknowledge that the training schools teach it conscientiously and carefully, but that it is not all we need to learn. What have we then learned, what have we heard, that goes deeper than these practical details? We have had many talks and addresses from the doctors; serious lectures these; often they are published and stand for future time. We must find something in them all, surely, to nourish our out-reaching aspirations?

Oh, these yearly recurring talks! One on every graduation day in every training school throughout the land! Let us be frank and admit plainly once for all that they are wearisome, perennial rubbish. These men who among themselves are so brilliant, so learned, so interesting, how can they—from which their brain-cells do they produce the thin, unflavored mental pabulum which they gravely serve out to us? And we, as we sit on the platform full of enthusiasm, how gladly would we hear something to stimulate and inspire us as thinking beings!

What do we really hear? Advice about squeaking shoes and rustling aprons; about washing up the dishes and not making work for the servants; about respecting the feelings of the family nurse and not contradicting the grandmother's prescriptions. What a relief it would be if some day we could rise in a body and, once for all, say, "Friend, we have been told all of this in the training school, and even if we had not, it would be too late now, for you to try to teach it." Fortunately for us we know that in reality these same men, the next day, would not recognize their own platitudes, and would almost to a man defend the nurse from the officious relative, and even stand by her though the dishes remained unwashed, providing she took the right care of the patient.

But what do they teach us of ethics? Well, this,— as yet the extremest that we have heard,—the nurse's whole duty, loyalty, and obedience begins and ends in subordination to the doctor. Beyond this there is no horizon and outside of this she has no reason for existing. Ponder over this dictum and acknowledge that there is something unsatisfying in it. No doubt here is involved a great ethical principle. May one know the whole, or only a part? Why is it put just so without any exception or alternative? Perhaps there is something more than this. One would like to see the nurse allowed the same amount of independence as any other moral being.

Suppose she were to be taught that her duty and loyalty were to be, first, to truth and justice as living principles. This understood, it becomes unnecessary to reiterate these cautions about being loyal to the doctor. Naturally she will be loyal to him; why not? Not only is it to her interest to be so, but, presumably, truth and justice will exact it, in nine cases out of ten. Yet it is quite possible to imagine that in the tenth case there might be circumstances which would make it wrong for her to obey and remain subordinate to the doctor, just as it might be wrong for a doctor to uphold the nurse. According to justice and truth, her loyalty might be due, not to the doctor, but to the patient. Or, not to either of these but to the patient's friends. Or, away from them all and to the public.

There is an obedience which is slavishness, and a subordination which is moral cowardice. But how is one to draw the line? It is a delicate subject, and requires a great deal of knowledge. True. It requires a knowledge of our obligations and duty to all classes of people, not only to one class.

Would we not, in a study of these obligations on all sides, find our ethics, and would not such study be more profitable than didactic regulations? How much new light would be thrown upon our own problems, and what fresh meaning appear in all branches of our own work!

As a class of working women, or professional women, or whatever we like to call ourselves, we nurses, taking us the world over, are deficient in this sort of knowledge. When one considers the character of our own special work our deficiency seems hardly to be accounted for.

In our own homes where everything was comfortable and our surroundings not very expansive we had no special occasion to wonder about such things. The little charities and works of benevolence in which we indulged, were, we were told, about all that was necessary or even advisable to do for other people. When, under the pressure of one impulse or another we entered the hospitals, we found a life in which the whole of everything was comprised under two heads; the patient, and the doctor. That was plain, easy, and satisfactory. We liked that. But now that we are out of the training schools we find ourselves in a vast world of duties and responsibilities of which we have scarcely heard a whisper. Shall we conclude that the training school has neglected our education, and that we have been imposed upon by not having all these things taught us while we were there? Before we think that, let us recall what it actually did do for us.

When we entered the hospital some of us had never made a bed; did not know the difference between the coffee-pot and the tea-kettle, and had never in our lives had to "tidy up" as we went along. Some of us had never borne a serious responsibility, had never been compelled to be on time. What easy-going habits of mind we had! Few had been trained to logical consecutive thinking. Accuracy was a sort of slavery; we resented it and loved to fall back into slip-shod ways. We had all kinds of dispositions, too,—were not always easily taught. It was easier sometimes to take offence than to accept a new idea.

When our head nurses, anxious to improve us, criticised our short comings, we imagined they had taken a wierd, fantastic dislike to us. By far the clearest and best thinking some of us did was on the subject of the faults of our superior officers, and there were few occasions when we could not have given our superintendent valuable points. How much we thought we knew, and how little we actually did know!

In those two years beside all our practical work we took courses in hygiene, anatomy, physiology, materia medica and cooking. We tried to absorb something of bacteriology, that vast subject to which men devote whole lives. We had to memorize somehow an entire dictionary of scientific terms in order to understand the speech of our chiefs. We had to learn something of hospital management; of household economy on a large scale.

Can we really think that we ought also to have been taught scientific ethics? Remember we had every example and opportunity in the elements of practical ethics. Can we complain that we were not broadened in social science? Compare the actual extent of two years time and the size of our brains with the full extent of all we had to learn, and no other answer will be needed. But we need not feel discouraged; rather rejoice in the thought that there is more to learn and more time in which to learn it. Because we are graduates we need not stand still, but rather carry on our post-graduate class work in our graduate associations. These are not meant only to be accident insurance companies (I mean no disrespect to sick benefit funds, which are among the first practical duties of our alumnae) but also schools in which the nurses' education may be continued. Was not this the leading motive of those broad-minded and far-seeing members of our craft who have worked to organize their school associations, and have not our overworked superintendents of training schools, weighted with the burden of all they have to do for their pupil's education, refreshed themselves with the thought that in encouraging these associations they were making the best provision for their graduates' future welfare? Heretofore everything has been done for the nurse. Now let her show what she can do for herself. In her training course, instruction was carefully prepared, brought and offered to her. Perhaps she did not always appreciate it as she might have done.

It is said that if chickens have all their food given to them without having to scratch for any of it, they become unhealthy. Maybe we, like chickens, will become sturdier by having to scratch for some of our own mental nourishment. There is no teacher like voluntary association, no means of developing character greater than that offered by associated life. If nurses do not realize this, they should observe the development of the average woman's club. It begins usually with self-culture, is literary, perhaps, rather timorous and quite exclusive. Presently it gets into the subject of general education, and before it knows where it is, it has become democratic, casts artificial social distinctions aside and is in the thick of public school work, public amusements, municipal housekeeping, public hygiene, the housing and condition of the poor, and, in short, the whole open world of its obligations and responsibilities to all people. Marvellous practical results, marvellous ethical influences flow from this little group, not the least wonderful of which is, that women who at first asked, "What good will this club be to me? What is there in this to benefit me?" are in a short while saying, "What is there in me for this club? What good can I be to my fellow-members?"

Of course, I do not mean that nurses can all go into public work. This is simply an illustration of what associated life can do. Have I ever been heard to say, "What good does my association do me? What do I get from it?" If so, set me down as self-convicted of being in the very first stages of ethical development. If I feel that I have nothing to get it is because I have not tried to give anything. There are about us beautiful examples of people who are constantly giving out to others, and, strange to say, the more they give out the more they seem to possess. This is said to be the real meaning of the old Bible words, "To him that hath shall more be given."

Of course, everyone knows that nurses are busy people, leading a laborious life, and not having much time to attend meetings or read. As for the meetings perhaps they might really get to them oftener if they were always interesting. The real reason meetings are often neglected is because they are dull. And who shall criticize? For, if you go and find your club or alumnae meeting dull, is it not, perhaps, your own fault?

There is too much "shop" in many of these meetings; too much careful anxiety over minute constitutional points and what might be called domestic affairs. Not but that these latter are important, only, they need not take up all the time; and as for the constitution,—oh! that it might be abolished altogether, and just a few simple and easily altered rules of procedure take its place. The constitution is intellectually a snare and practically a clog. Valuable time, yes, precious time, is often given to discussing it and tinkering at it, which ought to be spent on something worth while. If, after the domestic affairs are settled some broader line of study might be taken up in our gradute's association; some question which makes us feel that we are related also to the world of the living and the active! Those organizations of nurses are the most vigorous and successful which take up for consideration subjects of general interest and are thus brought into comradeship with busy, interesting people outside of their own work. As for the books. Well, of course, if we mean to study Greek we shall need books, but if, instead, we mean to study the question of our responsibilities to all people and our opportunities for helping to make the world a better, healthier, and happier place to live in, for others and also for ourselves, we do not need books. For this kind of study no one is more advantageously placed than we. Too busy to read books and study, we are busy right there in the world, where all the information we need to get is ready at first hand. Why study books when we can study life? We can make our own books. Between us all, what kinds of people, what kinds of life are there, that we do not learn to know? If I, for instance, only know the problems of the rich, you, in your different work, may understand everything about the life of the poor. If one has simply learned her responsibilities to the medical profession, another may be able to balance that one-sidedness by a knowledge of duties to other working women or to the cause of better education in general. We only need to exchange information, and, if, in our busy lives we come into contact with the people who are actually doing the things that books are written about, redressing grievances, extending freedom, pursuing justice, is not this better than books?

Our associations might be our store rooms and clearing houses, where everything should be brought together for the general good. We would find there, to our surprise, that others of whom we never even knew are affected, indirectly, perhaps, but still affected by what we do; and that many of our actions, to us, perhaps, comparatively unimportant, are of great importance in their relation to other people.

In studying our obligations to others we will incidentally learn what we owe to ourselves and each other. This, too, is something to which we have not given enough attention. Many plain working people have sounder and more intelligent ideas regarding their responsibilities to one another as fellow-workers, than have nurses, who have been heard to say that in their work they stood alone, that they owed nothing to others, and that they did not recognize the right of their fellow-members in the association to be concerned in their professional actions or to have anything to say to them in the way of advice or criticism; in a word, some among us hold the doctrine that what they do is of no concern to any one but themselves. This sort of idea shows what page of the primer they have reached and how much they have to learn. From working people who have gone farther ahead we will learn that when one enters any branch of active duty, let it be called trade, calling, profession, what one will, one inherits, as it were, all the accumulated advantages which have accrued through the labors of all the former workers; one takes at once a recognized standing and possesses certain privileges as the result of the striving of all who have gone before. It is, therefore, considered a clear case of shirking, only to be accounted for by ignorance or selfishness, when one declines to acknowledge any obligation in return, or refuses to recognize one's duty to those who will come after. Among the modern teachers and writers on this sort of question one occasionally meets the phrase "class-conscious," expressing the special knowledge which members of a working fraternity acquire in the study of their duties to one another, and nurses need to cultivate something of this "class-consciousness;" that is, they need to become better acquainted with the construction and conditions of their profession as a whole, and to make more of a study of its history, its status, its weak points, its aspirations, and its possibilities for the future.

Among the obligations we owe to ourselves and to each other comes before everything else, independence of outside control in our personal and professional affairs. This, too, is the first condition requisite for taking up the study of our social relations and opportunities. Undoubtedly, we nurses in America, are as compared with those of some other countries, quite free in our post-graduate life; yet even with us are still to be found nurses' associations which are almost entirely controlled by the medical societies, and others where the nurses' practical business, the registry, is managed by the boards of managers of training schools. Under such management the graduates have no voice in making rules or regulations, in selecting the executive officer, or in disposing of the income from registry fees. In short, instead of being domestic such registries are the sheerest oligarchies. Nurses who accept such conditions are greatly to be censured. They are ignoring the first duty of the inhabitants of a free country, namely, to *be* free, and though they may not wish freedom for themselves they should at least know that they have no moral right to make it more difficult of attainment for those who do care for it. By placing themselves permanently in a position of unnecessary and therefore belittling subordination (one would not say that *all* subordination was belittling), they hold back their whole class. Associations so hampered will never develop vigorously or go far in the study of their social responsibilities. Strange enough is it that a profession, noble as is that of our chiefs, and held as it is to be free from the commercial spirit, should ever be found willing to conduct small business enterprises such as nurse's registry, not scorning to apply to their medical libraries the modest income therefrom, which they have not earned, but which is contributed by one of the hardest working class of those who serve; but is not the attitude of these bands of women stranger? To know that they might stand independently, but that they prefer contributing to those who do not hesitate taking advantage of them? By far the large majority of the medical profession, as we all know, are too liberal and generous minded to think of establishing a commercial relation between themselves and nurses. They wish to see us thoroughly able, dignified, and self-respecting. Why, then, should we encourage the less considerate, by allowing them pecuniary advantages which the more thoughtful would not condescend to ask for? They are all alike our chiefs, and we owe them all the same fair, honorable dealing. Instead of that we show them partiality and special favors, the very opposite of what our duty demands from us. The same confusion is present in our financial relations with the training school management, and the principle of loyalty is so plausibly associated therewith as to befuddle the brains of many a young and true-hearted graduate.

As a matter of plain fact, the conduct of a registry has no bearing whatever on one's loyalty to one's school. A registry is simply a piece of business, planned for the purpose of making it easier for patients to get nurses and for nurses to receive their calls. It has absolutely no logical connection with training school work now, in our American system, and its survival here and there in this connection is simply a relic of the religious sisterhood days. As our graduate nurses are no longer a part of an institution, they should take over the control of their affairs from the institution. If there is care and responsibility it is theirs and they should bear it. There comes up, too, in these cases the question of the dues. What are they for? Naturally, to pay expenses, and, reasonably, to have a reserve on hand for the benefit of the women who earn them. But there is a surplus which goes toward training school expenses, and as no account of it is ever made to the graduates, and as they are never thanked for giving it, one can only infer that it is due to the school. Do we then owe the training school this money? We have never been told so, and if we were paying a debt it would in time be discharged.

Perhaps the training school is in need of money? Then it would be the right thing for us to pay for our tuition there. It is our Alma Mater and we love it very dearly; it has done great things for us and is doing them for others. How much sweeter, more gracious, and more rational of us to subscribe and give to it voluntarily as a thank-offering what we now give underhandedly in a muddled sort of way as registry dues! We could then attend to our own business and would not have this confusion of mind as to how much, in our motives, is loyalty, how much self-interest, and how much compulsion.

The graduates of men's and women's colleges and universities take a lively and practical interest in the affairs of their Alma Mater, its financial condition, its general policy, its advancement, its attitude on all questions of general importance, its changes or modification of curriculum. Are they more loyal than we? It would seem so. Or else, we succeed in combining deep loyalty with an equally great indifference, for to actively interest ourselves in these questions is the last and least thing that many of us would think of. We have not realized the great practical help, the great moral support, that we might be to our old school and its leaders, who perhaps, are constantly having to struggle single-handed to retain the advantages which we enjoyed, and to widen out the opportunities for the oncoming pupils. It is because we have not studied our responsibilities and obligations from an ethical standpoint. Perhaps, too, our school has not taken us enough into confidence, has, also, not realized the strength there might be in us, has not called upon us to rally to its support when some critical moment arrived in the slow progress towards shorter working hours, longer study time, less cramming, more careful preparation for a life of tremendous responsibility. How many of us have given more than a passing thought to the struggle, the strain endured by those of our fellow-members, who, in charge of training school work have won and now hold those advantages which we accept so easily and criticise so glibly? Why should they alone struggle for these objects? Why should we not help to attain them? Is it nothing to us if many nurses are overworked and undertaught; if the course is too short; the hours too long; if pupils are sent to private duty to earn money for the hospital, and if training school management is taken over by political, or by commercial hands? Is there not here something to bring before the consideration of our post-graduate associations?

A more thorough knowledge of training school problems is urgently advisable for the higher education of graduate nurses. At present they are, almost to a woman, deficient in such knowledge and, consequently, also deficient in the sympathy which they should feel toward those bearing the burdens. A better knowledge would bring the sympathy and would improve the quality of the loyalty by infusing intelligence therein. The Sisters of the Old World training schools, who are, it is true, in a position of subordination to an institution their lives long, yet have a personal interest in and knowledge of the affairs of the whole, and receive in turn the appeals and the confidence of the school with a completeness and unity too often lacking amongst us. In our graduate life as related to the training school we American nurses are, as yet, neither one thing nor the other. We have outgrown, naturally and rightly, the old form of lifelong dependence (though, what seems a pity, we have lost also much that was sweet and affectionate in this relation), and we have not yet arrived at the spontaneity of free, voluntary, enthusiastic support and interest shown by college graduates to their schools. We are, in this respect, a tame, colorless anomaly.

All these questions lead us back to the subject of our professional and ethical culture, and upon this depends our status in the community and our value professionally and socially. We all realize this, and the one question on which nurses most often express themselves is that of the competition of the ill-taught, half-equipped nurse. We are evidently in many ways a success, for every small hospital wants to have us; or, is it only that we are, as pupils, a money-saving device? Even in our probationer year we do an immense amount of work for considerably less cost to the hospital than the wages of untrained domestics would amount to, and we are an advertisement for the hospital. Many patients enter because the nurses are there who would not do so were they absent. Now, we must ask ourselves, why do we do this? Because we wish to get a special education. Very well; but suppose we all do this work and then after all do not get the education—only a smattering—enough to deceive ourselves and, to a certain extent, other people. Here, too, loyalty to a school or hospital needs to be illuminated by common sense. Can we inquire into our ethical responsibilities to other people without discovering theirs to us? Can we go far in applying a strict ethical standard to our own actions without demanding that we shall also find it in the actions of others toward us? If I treat you as I wish to be treated, equally true is it that you must treat me as you wish to be treated. Otherwise, you become an aggressor and I have soon lost my dignity and spirit and am imposed upon unfairly.

If we do the work in these hospitals we ought to receive the education. But many hospitals undertaking to train nurses are not fitted to give a complete education. Then, these, as has been often suggested by our leaders, should employ graduates or coöperate with other institutions, and women seeking a thorough education should shun them. These, naturally, will not have sufficient experience to judge, but a coördinated profession striving toward advancement might know; might make it a part of its most special responsibilities to others to advise and guide; might have distinct influence in supporting and encouraging the best teaching and in helping to solve the problem of the special hospital in some way which should be as much to the interest of the hospital as the present plan, and which should also be what the present unregulated system of small training schools is *not*, industrially just and educationally righteous. These two lines, the industrial and the educational, need to be studied together. We are familiar with the latter. The former is not so well known to us, but if we should enter upon some study of general industrial questions as an approach to our own work, we would find it, not only of the most absorbing interest, capable of inspiring an enthusiasm hitherto unknown among us, but also the most instructive and enlightening possible, clearing up a hundred misty points and supplying us with examples and lessons illustrative of every difficulty and its remedy.

Shall we learn self expression in the future? In the past we have been a silent Sisterhood. It would seem as if we had had little to say to one another. Yet people of common interests are usually never done communicating with each other; they fill magazines, write, talk, even telegraph their latest discoveries or purposes. But we have heretofore stood aloof, looked askance, and spoken in monosyllables. True, the work of a nurse is depressing, repressing, and very confining. Yet if the whole truth were told it would have to be confessed that as a profession we have not had sense of unity until very lately. Even yet it is somewhat feeble and needs much cultivation, and if our work tends to separate us from one another and from the stimulating and invigorating things of life, we ought consciously and deliberately to put forth every effort to counteract and minimize this tendency. One can hardly agree with the criticism often heard and read, that the discipline of the training school ruins individuality, and that the obedience one works under there makes one dull, for one sees so many characters develop finely and unexpectedly under that discipline and grow in self-reliance, fortitude and judgment. But we do need to give much thought to this question of the true development of the well-poised individual, for, with our opportunities for free self-government, if we remain stultified and half-grown it can be the fault of no one but ourselves. True, we must often obey, but it is only obedience for the sake of obedience, or for a worthless cause, that deteriorates character. If one were to submit to wind spools forever without knowing what the spools were for, one would grow dull, but with such work as ours, intelligently understood, the necessary obedience is only the harmony and order by which all may be accomplished. It is only, like our old friend etiquette, a preventive of friction, not a principle of ethics. For our own balance and safety we need to study attentively the relation between the individual and the work. Which is most important? If the work is most important then it would be right that the individual should be sacrificed or practically subordinated; if the individual is most important, then the work must suffer. If, however, they are each, in their own way and at their own times, equally important, then we must learn how to recognize, at the right time, the supremacy of the work, and how to insist, also at the right time, upon the supremacy of the individual. The sensible way to regard obedience is as a part of the uniform, to be put on for the clean, thorough, successful accomplishment of a definite piece of work; and taken off with the uniform when that piece of definite work is done. If we wear uniform all the time, we find presently that it has created for us a set of artificial distinctions through which we cannot easily break, and surely if we adopt obedience as a law for the soul it will stand in our way and bar every turn toward progress. We need not to condemn or discard rational and purposeful obedience, but to avoid the pointless and uncalled for obedience and tractability to others in general affairs which are of mental laziness, and which prevent initiative, independent thought, and self-reliant action.

The wonderful thing about the study of ethics, one's relation to others, is that it has no end. It expands indefinitely as we go forward in it. As the conscience of the moral man, yesterday, would not permit him to be cruel to a slave, and to-day will not allow him to have a slave, and, perhaps, to-morrow, will not let him rest until that slave stands on a level with himself, so will our consciences not allow us to remain contented, to-day, with the little duties which yesterday satisfied us, and to-morrow our aspirations and endeavors for the good of all will go far ahead of what we see to-day. Our obligations were yesterday to ourselves; to-day, they are to our classmates; to-morrow they will be to all human beings. But if, in a prosaic and perhaps somewhat sordid round of bread-and-butter earning we allow ourselves to lose our imagination, we may miss, for many years to come, this normal growth and remain stunted and ill-developed.

"Hospital Organization"

In the rapidly proliferating hospitals of the early 1900s, the authority system was shifting. Here the National Hospital Record (6 [1903]: 10-14) gave Lavinia Dock the opportunity to present organized nursing's viewpoint on the training school superintendent's place in the hospital hierarchy.

Clearly Dock and Lillian Wald believed that having the training school superintendent report directly to the trustees would enhance her authority. From today's perspective we can see that the two women were looking backward to nineteenth-century social structures. The twentieth century would see the trustees, with their traditional philathropic outlook, yield power to the medical staff, the new men of science.

Hospital Organization.

BY MISS L. L. DOCK.

WITHIN the last year or so several papers, with subsequent discussions, have appeared on the subject of hospital organization,[1] and as regards the training school and nursing work which forms a part of every hospital of importance these contributions show so inadequate a grasp of the relation of what one paper calls the "women folks" to the whole that it may not be out of place to consider the views advanced thereon from the standpoint of the said "folks."

Dr. Smith writes: *"The superintendent of the hospital should be appointed by the Medical Board with the approval of the managers. * * * The term of service of the superintendent should be three years, but he should be eligible for reappointment. The matron should be the superintendent of the training school for nurses, and after the first class has graduated, she should be selected by the medical board*[2] *by preference from the list of graduates of the school and approved by the managers. The term of service of matron should be* FIVE *years, but she should be eligible for reappointment.*

"In the organization of the training school the medical board should exercise full authority under the managers. It should prescribe rules and regulations governing the school, arrange the course of instruction, select the instructors, appoint the superintendent of the training school and examine the candidates for graduation."[3]

This plan, it will be seen, gives the trustees little or no real share in the hospital management beyond the appointing of the medical board, and presumably the supplying of necessary funds. How this arrangement would personally affect the superintendent of a hospital I will leave him to say. Certainly it would leave the superintendent of nurses without firm ground under her feet when nurses had to be changed for training, or when unlimited "specials" were demanded, and under such a system nurses and nursing would quickly revert to a former type, of which survivals may be seen to-day in those Austrian and French hospitals where the entire control of nursing arrangements is in the hands of the medical staff. Dr. Smith is right in unifying the work of matronship with nursing, and he also is right in quoting Miss Nightingale's dictum[4] that the discipline of the nurses should be left entirely to the head of nurses; he, however, fails to see that under his plan of organization this possibility would be entirely destroyed.

Dr. Rowe, who is one of the most notable executives to be found in hospitals, gives quite a different picture of the relationship proper between trustees, medical staff and hospital superintendent. He is strong in his ideas of organization and discipline on what may be called the side of the men, but weak in those affecting the women of the hospital. While he describes the trustees or board of managers as the ultimate source of power, yet

---

[1] Report of the Committee on Hospitals, Dispensaries and Nursing, Stephen Smith, M. D., chairman, read at the Second New York State Conference of Charities and Corrections.

[2] "Observations on Hospital Organization," by George H. M. Rowe, M. D., read at the fourth annual meeting of the National Association of Hospital Superintendents.

[3] The italics are mine.

[4] At the time this paper was read, Miss Lillian D. Wald, head of the Nurses' Settlement, New York City, and a member of the committee on "Hospitals, Dispensaries and Nursing," submitted the following minority report, which has been incorporated in the proceedings of the conference:
Miss Wald takes exception to that portion of the report which recommended that a superintendent of nurses be selected from the graduates of the school, and that such superintendent be appointed by the medical board. Miss Wald thus states her objection:
Selection of superintendents of nurses from graduates of the school.—While this may often be the most successful plan, yet it cannot be stated as a fixed principle. Its disadvantage is that it tends to narrowness, and the best development of the school is often attained by bringing in from the outside a head who may infuse fresh vitality and bring new ideas into the life of the school.
The superintendent of nurses.—First, her appointment by the medical board. This might also work well in individual cases, but the principle is wrong. The superintendent of nurses is one of the most important administrative officers of the hospital, and her selection

so far as the women's departments are concerned he would have this but a power in the abstract. He says:

"The trustees should choose the executive officers and control the appointment of other officers:—naturally, an unpaid board of busy men in a large hospital must rely on the superintendent to investigate the fitness of applicants for positions, *even depending upon him to nominate** the more important ones, such as * * * *matron, superintendent of the training school,* * * * etc." And again, "He should take charge of the general management of all the affairs of the hospital, except the professional care of the patients. * * * He should *select the officers,** employes, and servants of every grade." * * *

Later he speaks with disapprobation of the trustees appointing the superintendent of nurses, and making her responsible to themselves, his criticism being that this places her "*outside the jurisdiction of the superintendent.*"

In the discussion that followed this paper another hospital superintendent remarked: "That brings us back to the point of whether the head of the training school should be responsible to a committee of the board of managers, or should be responsible to the superintendent of the hospital. The superintendent of the hospital, if he be a fair man, needs to be supported by his managers; he should be responsible to that board of managers and every head of the different departments should be responsible to him as the executive officer of that board.

Another said: "He (the superintendent) has absolute authority in the administration of the affairs of the hospital. He does not interfere with the treatment of patients, but * * * . *Under him are superintendent of nurses and a matron.*"

This subordination of the chief woman executive is what Dr. Rowe calls the "unal" plan.

The term "unal" is obviously misleading, and inaccurately used, for it is at once evident that, since the medical staff is left out, it does not cover the entire hospital organization.

The above quotations all specifically mention the medical portion of the hospital work and the medical set of hospital officials as not coming under the full control of the hospital superintendent, and completely "unal" control is therefore not in question. Need it follow that disorder will result? Not at all, for the superintendent of the hospital has the power given him by the trustees to hold a check over all parts of the hospital work, by which he may preserve the equilibrium of the whole. Dr. Rowe's use of the word "unal" really signifies the subordination of the training school part of the work.

Would equality of position for the training school superintendent—always bearing in mind that in points relating directly to the

---

is as much the rightful privilege of the trustees of the hospital as that of the superintendent.

The superintendent of nurses has a threefold responsibility: 1. To the managers of the hospital on the side of household economy and harmonious ordering of the domestic side of ward work. Also for the reputation of the training school with the public, that it may have the confidence of patients, and attract a high class of women nurses. 2. To the medical staff for the performance of orders and treatment of the sick. 3. To the women who enter the school and to their friends and families not only for their proper education, but also that they are protected and given due position and consideration.

A superintendent of nurses appointed by the medical board will almost inevitably overdo her responsibility to them and slight her other two equally great responsibilities.

While theoretically the interests of all are identical, in practical details one set of interests will crowd the others, unless the superintendent of nurses is a balance wheel to preserve all in a due state of equilibrium.

Examples.—The medical board may require her to supply special nurses to pay-patients, *The italics are mine.

beyond her capacity, thus understaffing the free wards; or they may ask for special nurses for free cases beyond the number which the hospital is financially able to support; or in many ways may so add to the clerical and serving work of the nurses, as to make a staff which ought to be quite adequate for all nursing work practically insufficient; to such demands the superintendent of nurses must be able to say "no," with the sense that she is also to guard the interests of the trustees, and that they will uphold her.

Her appointment for five years.—This, if practiced, would have most unfortunate results. The best woman would refuse the position under such a condition. As the end of her term approached, her duties would be neglected and her attention distracted by the wish for reappointment; she would cultivate those with influence; would learn to pull wires, to be unduly subservient, and the whole atmosphere of political jobbery would be introduced. If not actually working for reappointment she would be suspected of doing so, and her subordinates would lose her confidence in her motives. She should be appointed during satisfactory service, and dismissed at any time when the interests of the school required.

hospital as a whole she will necessarily defer to him—mean "dual" control? Even if it did, it might be proper to modify views such as were quoted above, for after all, what is a hospital? It is simply a large family, as Dr. Rowe also calls it, resting upon a basis of housekeeping and presenting in an extreme form all the problems of the family.

The orthodox conception of the family, in many countries and many centuries, was of course on the "unal" plan, the man being the unit. But modern states are abolishing by legislation this "unal" form and are replacing it by a dual constitution of the family. The woman has long had equal property rights, and she is now becoming equal guardian of her children. With the disappearance of patriarchalism the modern family is seen to have two heads—on the principle, I suppose, that two heads are better than one. However, in hospitals, I stanchly advocate having one head. Work goes much better so, and this one I take to be, by rights, by logic and by common sense, the trustees or managers, whatever their corporate name may be. Nor would I have this leadership an abstract or academic thing, but a practical working authority.

There can be no doubt whatever that the trustees are really the head of the hospital. The superintendent might be removed, and the hospital might, conceivably, still run on, after a fashion. The superintendent of the training school might be eliminated, but the hospital would still continue. Even the medical board might go, and the hospital need not cease to exist. But remove the trustees finally and irrevocably and the hospital comes to an end.

The trustees thus being the true source of power, why should they not appoint the superintendent of nurses, who is undeniably an important executive officer, and make her responsible to themselves?

In the minds of the large majority, as I believe, of nurses who have had hospital experience, there is every reason , why they should do so, and no reason why they should not. One might except hospitals of small or medium size having a trained nurse in the position of hospital superintendent. Even in such cases, should the hospital grow large and administration complex, it would be the proper system to make the superintendent of nurses responsible to the trustees, as the woman who was strong as a financier and general executive might be, and very possibly would be, less interested in the teaching side, and therefore should not be allowed the possibility of hampering or restricting that most important branch of the service.

The basis of this feeling among hospital women is, that ward management and nurse training are becoming such highly developed and many-sided pieces of expert work that they are rising entirely out of the position of "subordinate departments" which Dr. Rowe assigns them.

Indeed, it seems as if the entire organization plan of a great hospital should be grouped in larger sections, and that some new technical terms should be introduced into it to describe such sections. It might, for instance, be considered that a large hospital, or even one of moderate size, was made up of three sections, each section being composed of numerous departments, and each department

---

EXTRACTS FROM THE REPORT OF THE ENGLISH HOSPITAL COMMISSION, 1900.

*The "suggestions" printed in Appendix K to the first volume of the evidence show clearly what are Miss Nightingale's views on this subject. She says: "The superintendent (i. e., matron) should herself be responsible to the constitutional hospital authorities, and all her nurses and servants should, in the performance of these duties, be responsible to the superintendent only. No good ever comes of the constituted authorities placing themselves in the office which they have sanctioned her occupying. No good ever comes of any one interfering between the head of the nursing establishment and her nurses. It is fatal to discipline. She should be made responsible for her results and not for her methods. Of course, if she does not exercise the authority intrusted to her with judgment and discretion, 't is then the legitimate province of the governing body to interfere, and to remove her. It is necessary to dwell strongly on this point, because there has been not unfrequently a disposition shown to make the nursing establishment responsible on the side of discipline to the medical officer or the governor of the hospital. Neither the medical officer nor any other male head should ever have power to punish for disobedience. His duty should end with reporting the case to the female head who, as already stated, is to the government of the infirmary alone, for efficient discharge of her duties." The opinion thus expressed by Miss Nightingale appears (so far as the evidence shows), to be generally adopted in the metropolitan hospitals, both (as already stated) by the medical staff and also by the governing authorities themselves.

consisting of several or many sub-departments, and so finally coming down to the individual workers. They might be so arranged:

Section 1.—That part belonging to the physicians and surgeons. This could, surely, only be most improperly called a department of the hospital, and it is usually divided into a considerable number of departments.

Section 2.—The business part of the hospital, including all that is usually looked upon as the man's share of family responsibility, viz.: the providing of supplies, maintenance, renovation, finance, with all the departments and sub-departments coming under such classification.

Section 3.—All that part usually described as 'woman's work" viz.: the utilization of supplies, housekeeping, home-making, teaching, nursing.

While this distinction between men's and women's work is not at all scientific, it follows the usual custom of modern hospitals, and even supposing that hospitals were conducted entirely by men, or entirely by women, this is the logical division of work and responsibility. As an actual fact, it is the failure of men in general to understand or to *practically* recognize women's work, and the quite common failure of hospital superintendents and the medical staff to comprehend the province of the superintendent of nurses, that is at the bottom of most of the "friction" found in hospitals.

In a business, or in a home, or in a hospital, where every one has a complete understanding of the duties, the responsibilities, and the rights of all the others, friction will be minimized.

For what is "friction?" It is an effort toward adjustment; it is the protest of the disorganized and unsystematized.

In a disorderly business, or home, or hospital, where no one knows exactly what another one ought to do or has the right to do, there *ought* to be friction, for otherwise there would be dull acquiescence in all sorts of improper arrangements—one of the worst of conditions.

Dr. Rowe speaks wisely when he advocates placing the matronship and the training school work under one head. They belong together, and to separate them is like setting the sides of the body in opposition. Under different heads, the matrons' ideal is to conserve her stores;—the nurses' to use them up. Even the best of nurses are inconsiderate toward the laundry and linen room until the weight of responsibility for these portions of the hospital whole is brought home to them. The kitchen also belongs to this division, although I am quite well aware that as yet few superintendents of nurses are ready to take it. Nevertheless this is its logical and proper place. I do not forget, either, that it is quite possible to have good results with the right people under a poor system, and poor results with the wrong people under a good system. But if the system is upon the right lines and a sound foundation then one has the best reason for hoping to find the right individuals. Let us examine Section 3 a little more closely to see of what it consists.

Dep't. 1.—The housekeeping of the wards and of the entire house, including the engaging and managing of maids.

Dep't. 2.—The laundry, with all its service and records.

Dep't. 3.—The linen rooms and supply rooms, including the book-keeping incidental to this part of work.

Dep't. 4.—The sustenance of the patients and of the entire family, including the management of the kitchen, special diet kitchens, cooking lessons, the purchasing of food supplies and the account keeping of the same, or else the requisitioning of the needed supplies.

Dep't. 5.—The nursing of patients, including the engaging and employment of orderlies, the requisitioning and preparation of surgical supplies, and the book and record keeping involved.

Dep't. 6.—The conduct of a school where the character of the pupils is peculiarly important, where technical training must be practiced upon human beings and where the standard of theoretical teaching is constantly rising. Add to this, that the responsibility of this school to the public is of a most serious and special nature; perhaps even beyond that of the medical school, necessitating discipline of a rigidly ethical kind.

Is it to be wondered at that a woman, or let us say a person, (for I am not contending for the rights of a woman, but for the right method of conducting a piece of work) prepared by special training and experience, and who is charged even with departments 5 and 6, and part of department No. 1, should feel that she is hampered and handicapped, if she is not able to present her problems and her budget directly to the trustees, who are the final power? She cannot often feel sure that the superintendent of the hospital understands all of her work well enough to represent it for her, or to direct it through her. Nor, if she is in this irrationally subordinate position, does she always feel free to develop her initiative. It may be said, "Will she be any better off with the trustees?" At least she will have the same opportunity the hospital superintendent feels so important for himself, that of educating them, and they will be likely to treat her, if she is the right woman, as he wishes himself to be treated, namely, to agree with her as to general lines, leaving her the details.

May it be said: "Can she not hold this relation to the hospital superintendent with equally good results?"

No, for he does not possess the final power. He must go to the trustees himself, and if, overburdened with his own claims and problems, her's are lost in the transition, who can wonder?

Dr. Rowe regards this system with such disfavor that he asks: "Is not such a system illogical, unbusinesslike, conducive to friction, shifting the various responsibilities, subversive of the best discipline and tending to disrupt the household family?"

Fortunately, it is not necessary to argue this question from an academic standpoint, for there are concrete examples of hospitals established on this basis.

What are the actual facts? The hospitals having this plan of organization are conspicuously distinguished by good management, good discipline, absence of friction (comparatively speaking), definite placing of responsibility, and last but not least, by a quite noticeable atmosphere of cordiality and courtesy. Why not, when each one has respect for the other's position? In such hospitals the matron and principal would be more likely to go freely to the superintendent for consultation than under the "unal" plan. But there are other significant facts to be noticed in connection with this organization plan. Within the last few years we have seen several long established institutions change their system from the plan which Dr. Rowe advocates, to the one which he criticises. Why? Because their nursing was stationary, and because they could not induce the women they wanted to submit to subordination which would prevent progress. It would also be easy to mention hospitals which have failed to secure the women they would have liked to engage for teaching work, because they were not yet prepared to abandon these autocratic ideas as to the position of a training school superintendent.

I have known, for instance, of a hospital superintendent who hampered to such an extent his superintendent of nurses, that she was obliged to spend time in carrying pins around to the wards, which she should, instead, have given to reorganizing and supervising the nursing service. In this hospital the pupil night nurses were required to go in person to the doctor's rooms to report.

The regard of the well-trained nurse for her own profession, and for her professional chiefs, the medical men, is such that she desires for herself a truly dignified position, believing that she will thus best honor her own state, and best deserve the regard of the medical profession. Beside, it is, I believe, the duty of boards of trustees to be personally familiar with all the details of the work for which they are responsible to the public, and this is impossible unless they personally assume those direct relations with the heads of hospital sections which bring them into close touch with all sides of the hospital work.

"An Experiment in Contagious Nursing"

Published in Charities (11 [July 4, 1903]: 19-23), the leading social work journal of the day, this account gives a vivid picture of tenement life as the Henry Street visiting nurses saw it. Dock also describes municipal public health strategies at a time when infectious disease was the greatest threat to the nation's health--strategies with which the settlement nurses were closely involved.

An Experiment in Contagious Nursing
L. L. Dock,
Henry Street Nurses' Settlement, New York

The older members of the nursing staff of the Nurses' Settlement in Henry street have long been troubled by the question of contagion in the tenements. As a rule, contagious diseases are strictly banned by all district nursing associations. Those having printed rules usually state that the nurses will not be sent to contagious cases. We, having no printed rules and only such as are made by common assent, have always been rather more flexible in the matter of attending contagions than any other district nursing association that I know of, and have occasionally taken up some special case when the call was urgent. The conditions of excessive crowding in our neighborhood make complete isolation of contagious cases so absolutely impossible, that it often seemed more reprehensible to refuse some serious case than to disregard the principles of technique which, important as they are, are in practice almost grotesquely remote from the life about us. As we do not take obstetrical cases at all, it was usually possible to make some emergency arrangement.

In February last, it so happened that one nurse's services could be given entirely to this class of cases, and we decided to make an experiment which we hoped might be a demonstration and, perhaps, lead to some thoroughgoing system of oversight for these cases, Miss Hitchcock and I having visions of the free dispensaries establishing a nursing service for contagions, but Miss Wald already discerning the possibilities of municipal oversight through an extension of the functions of the Department of Health. During past administrations, when bad politics ruled, the contagious hospitals of the city were seriously neglected; more so even than other institutions, as they were less in the public eye. The Willard Parker Hospital, where the diphtheria cases were sent, was painfully inadequate in size, though the medical and nursing care were good. On North Brother's Island, a good scarlet fever pavilion was also absurdly small in bed space, and other wards were opened in decayed and brokendown shanties which a good, thrifty farmer would hardly have used for live stock.

The city of London provides hospital accommodation for seventy-five per cent of its contagious cases.

The city of New York, up to 1901, had

bed space for seven per cent. These figures speak for themselves.

When Dr. Ernst J. Lederle, the present health commissioner, took charge, the better handling of contagions from all sides, both in the hospital and in the homes, was one of the many reformations to which he devoted himself. His work beginning at the top, and ours going on at the bottom, were not long in meeting and the nursing care of contagions in crowded tenement quarters soon proved itself to be but one part of the whole great problem of municipal sanitation, not to be dealt with in a sporadic way, but as part of an orderly and comprehensive plan.

In many ways these are the neediest cases a district nurse can find. For one thing, the mothers, always nerveless and weak-hearted when it is a question of applying any treament against the resistance of a child, are doubly ineffective when the orders call for treatment so distinctly repugnant as nasal irrigation, throat spraying, and the like. The child violently resists, and few mothers can even hold the hands still except under the sternest mandates. The nurse quickly finds that, with rare exceptions, such orders are never carried out except when she is present. The fear of bathing and of air, so deeply grounded, it would appear, in European medical teaching, is universal among our foreign people, and it is a piteous sight to come into a small, stuffy, crowded room, with every window tightly closed, and find a child blazing with scarlet, or measles, with inflamed eyes, occluded nostrils, and angry throat, pasty and sticky with the dirt of a week upon him, and dressed in full woolen clothing, shoes and stockings, and an enormous scarf or towel swathed around his poor little neck, with probably a slice of greasy bacon tied underneath. The bed is invariably filthy, for the parents are afraid to annoy him. The stereotyped answer of the mother when the nurse asks whether this or that has been done is, "He won't let me." But especially is it from the larger standpoint of the family and the neighborhood that contagions are most serious. For the protection of the school, quite rightly, the well children are all excluded when there is a case of scarlet, measles or diphtheria at home. It is then at once evident what a large proportion of schooltime is thus lost by the children of the wage-earners of a great city, when one adds up the ten days to two weeks of measles, the ten days to four weeks of diphtheria, and the six to eight weeks of scarlet, during which the infection remains active.

Then, right beside this guarding of the schools and loss of schooltime to the well children, and in almost ludicrous contrast to it, goes on the crowded family life of the tenements, full of the most absurd details of "mixing up" sick and well in one vast and hopeless jumble. The father goes daily to his work whatever it may be, the older boys and young women go to their shops and factories, the mother goes daily to the market, jostles her neighbors on the stairs and stands in groups of adults with, as we have often seen, the infectious discharge from her child's nose or throat drying upon her apron. The friendly women of the same floor come in and sit about. Icemen and other vendors come and go. The old Hebrew teacher brings his smudgy books and sits beside the sick child's bed to teach the others their lessons. Pillows and bedding are indiscriminately used, blankets and sheets are shaken from the windows and aired on the fire-escapes.

The supervision of the Department of Health is as complete and strict as is possible under the circumstances. Physicians are required to report all contagious cases immediately, and an officer placards the door with a large card stating the disease within, and warning all against entrance. Leaflets in several languages are distributed, giving the clearest and most explicit directions for domestic disinfection.

Though, among the Jews, these leaflets are usually read, the conditions of the tenement are such that they are rarely followed, and I doubt if the Italians ever dream of paying any attention to them. They are usually found behind the looking-glass, or placed as a mat under the medicine bottles. In all throat cases cultures are taken, and antitoxin is furnished free, and is also administered by a physician from the department in response to calls from any part of the city, and with wonderful celerity. A

An Experiment in Contagious Nursing

medical inspector visits each contagious case once a week to watch progress and order disinfection, and this weekly visit is made with unfailing regularity. When the case terminates the rooms are disinfected, mattresses and bedding will be steam sterilized without cost, and the landlord is directed to clean and paint.

Yet with all this care and detail, isolation in the tenements is little more than a farce. For instance, Mrs. Doolan will meet the nurse thus: "Oh, the doctor from the board of health was round, and Johnny was playing in the entry with the boys, and the doctor was awful mad." (Johnny being in the "peelingest" stage of scarlet.)

Compulsory hospital service seems a necessity so fundamental, where people are so closely crowded together, that without it, inspection seems to a great extent a waste of time and trouble. If the hospitals were adequate, and the people were taught to understand that contagious diseases from crowded houses had to be sent there, they would soon become accustomed to the idea, and familiarity with the beneficial results of the hospital, when patients were sent early, would soon become a matter of general knowledge. As it is, the patients are often sent too late, when the parents are desperate, or when the patients are really almost in a dying condition. This is unfair to the hospital, and gives it, in many instances, a reputation among the poor as a place to be dreaded—a reputation which it does not deserve.

A feature of the work that gave me much concern was the frequency of nephritic complication in scarlet, and I felt certain that the nephritis I saw would not have occurred had the patients gone early to the hospital. The mothers feed the children too soon with solids, let them run about too soon, and do not give them enough fluid. Since the use of antitoxin, diphtheria has lost much of its terror, and is really less dreadful in the tenements than scarlet. Measles seems often a simple disease, yet no full evidence is at hand to show how many children recuperate fully in strength after it.

A difficult thing to combat is the prevalent belief that all children must have contagions. "What's the use of that," said one doubting father, who was a very intelligent man otherwise, "all children must have these sicknesses."

"Why, no," said the nurse, "I have never had them."

"Well, you will have them," replied the parent in tones of conviction.

Three months of this service, interesting as it was, was gladly given up by the settlement when it was found that the Department of Health was prepared to take it up. Dr. Lederle, already planning for extended hospital buildings and compulsory hospital service when the public health demanded it, established three nurses on the first of June to conduct a district nursing service for the contagious cases reported from the tenements of a definite manageable limit.

Mrs. Martha Peltier, a graduate of the New York City Hospital, took the diphtheria cases; Miss Katherine McNamara, of a Chicago hospital, was put on the scarlet fever cases, and Miss Katherine Healy, of the Kings County Hospital, Brooklyn, on the measles cases. They came to us a few days previously for initiation into the mysteries of streets, courts and houses and the preliminary supplies, and during June have reported every day at the settlement, their cases being telephoned down from the Health Department. They have used the bedside notes and daily records used in the settlement, and Miss Hitchcock, who has charge of all the nursing, has planned out with them their daily work, and has also assisted the department in arranging a very satisfactory mode of procedure for their technique in disinfection.

Dr. Lederle has now rented a small house next to the Willard Parker Hospital, and has cleaned it thoroughly and painted it throughout with enamel paint. The nurses live in their own quarters, but hereafter will come every morning in street dress to the little house. Here they change to their nursing uniform, and, returning in the late afternoon, again change, leaving off all external clothing, including boots, wraps and nursing bags. These are all carried in suitable receptacles to the disinfecting plant of the hospital, where they are sterilized over night, and returned early in the morning. The nurses now get their supplies from the hospital and will now no longer report at the settlement, but will continue to work as a district branch of the Health Department. Dr. Bryant of the Willard Parker Hospital has shown the greatest interest in the plan and has taken much pains to perfect the details relating to the co-operation of the hospital.

A schedule of the cases of three months is appended, with descriptions of a few typical family conditions.

The family of L—— lived in a very old and dilapidated rear tenement containing ten apartments of two small rooms each. ("Rear tenement" means that the house stands on the back of the lot and separated from the larger front house by about twelve or fifteen paces. In the little yard stands the row of horrible wooden privies where all discharges must be carried, unless they are emptied into the sink). Two families live on a floor, each having two rooms. The front one is sitting-room, kitchen, and laundry all in one, with an old couch or sofa where one person may sleep. The small room opening from it, with a little window at the back, is the bedroom, and holds one large bed with a pile of extra pillows. The L——s are father, mother, and five young children. No water supply is in the rooms, but must be carried from the landing in the entry. Here two children had a severe scarlet, and, while still ill, two others came down with measles.

Mrs. D—— lived in a similar apartment in a house equally wretched and

A SCHEDULE FOR THREE MONTHS.

Measles, 37 cases. { Complicated with pneumonia, 3.
" " glandular abscess, 1.
Simple uncomplicated cases, 28.

Diphtheria, 13 cases {
had antitoxin, 8. All recovered. { No complications, 7.
Glandular abscess, 1.
True cases but mild, 4.

Not considered true case, 1. As this case developed a typical septic rheumatism it was believed by the doctor in charge to be a true case, although the specific bacillus was not found.

Scarlet, 56 cases. {
Scarlet with inflammation and suppuration of ears, 3.

Scarlet with whooping cough, 1.

Scarlet with pneumonia, 1.

Scarlet of mediocre character with violent recurrence two weeks after first attack; intense purpuric confluent rash, and throat greatly swollen but without exudate. No complications or sequelæ. Recovery. 1.

Scarlet sent to hospital, 7. All did well.

Simple scarlet with no complications; throats red and tender but no exudate; no sequelæ up to time of fumigation, 25.

Violent scarlet with intense rash and severe symptoms; swollen glands and badly swollen throats and tongues. These cases all died in from one to seven days after the onset. 4

Complicated with diphtheria, 5. { Had antitoxin ; not enough, or too late— all died, 3.
No antitoxin, 2. { Recovered, 1.
Died, 1.

Simple scarlet with nephritis as sequel. In these all symptoms were mild; nephritis came on in one to three weeks after fading of rash, and lasted from one to four weeks, 3.

Scarlet with severe exudate on tonsils and { Inflammation of ear, 2.
with nephritis, 6; also of these five { Swollen glands, 2.
had further complications as shown. { Pneumonia, 1.

even airtier. She had five children, three of whom came down at the same time with scarlet. Although the medical inspector advised hospital she refused to let them go. However, as she was a widow, and largely dependent on charitable aid it was possible finally to compel her to send them.

The family W—— lived in a basement so far below the level of the street that it just did not come within the definition of a cellar. Their rooms were at the back, looking out upon a small courtyard, the level of which was almost to the top of their window. The living-room was dimly light, and the two bedrooms almost entirely dark. No sun ever reached any of the three. A case of scarlet here, strange to say, did well, and did not spread.

The Y—— family lived in three tiny rooms, fairly light, with seven children. Of these, three had measles, one had pneumonia, and one meningitis at the same time. The latter was sent to hospital, but the others remained at home, the parents, in the intervals of nursing, being engaged in selling white goods from a push-cart. The goods, which usually lay in the rooms at night, were kept down stairs while the children were ill, as the parents knew the Health Department would not allow them to be carried out of the room.

The K—— family were intelligent, and when two children came down with scarlet, they sent them at once to the hospital. While the department fumigated, the family sat upon the stairs for want of other place to go. Here the nurse found them and discovered that another little boy had the scarlet rash full out, and temperature of 104. They could not return to their rooms, so the ambulance was called and the patient carried off within half an hour.

"Some Urgent Social Claims"

In this address to the Nurses' Associated Alumnae in 1907 (<u>American Journal of Nursing</u> 7: 895-905), Lavinia Dock for the first time publicly appealed to her sister nurses to support women's suffrage. This year was a turning point in Dock's life. It saw the publication, to great acclaim, of the two-volume <u>History of Nursing</u>, which ranged from prehistoric times to the founding of the first American training schools. (The <u>History</u> is available in most libraries.) This was in a sense the climax of her work in nursing.

Also in 1907 the American suffrage movement, for some years dormant, came back to life with the founding in New York of the Equality League of Self-Supporting Women. The League's moving spirit, Harriot Stanton Blatch, daughter of the great woman's rights pioneer Elizabeth Cady Stanton, welcomed women of the working class and borrowed some of the flamboyant tactics of the British feminists. Lavinia Dock became a staunch adherent and one of Blatch's lieutenants. With political rights, Dock told the Associated Alumnae, they and other women could do much to relieve the plight of women and child laborers in industry. There was little response to her plea; one wonders how many nurses of the day had the energy or leisure for feminist or other concerns beyond their own bread and butter. The Alumnae, by then the American Nurses Association, endorsed women's suffrage in 1912; the constitutional amendment giving women the vote was passed in 1919 and ratified in 1920.

SOME URGENT SOCIAL CLAIMS

By L. L. DOCK

It is a long time since I have had the pleasure or privilege of meeting this society, and now that the opportunity has been given me, I am seizing it to speak to you on a subject which is not strictly in the line of our profession but which presses itself upon me, has always since I began to think about anything and every year more urgently, as the thing of all others which is of the nature of the next step; essential to the whole scope and reach of social progress and important in its bearing upon character development as well as a thing of concrete, practical possibilities in all work and all advance. I mean the subject of the political enfranchisement of women, which embraces the whole consideration of the many fields in which women are striving for a secure foothold, that they may live and express themselves and share those rights of life, liberty, and the pursuit of happiness which Thomas Jefferson declared to be inalienable. There are a number of reasons why I wished for permission to speak to you on this theme. One is, that I surmise to the majority of nurses it is a far-off, abstract, uninteresting theme, or even, it may be to some, one to be avoided with disapproval, or with the indifference of the extreme specialist toward all outside of a specialty. Another is that I am ardently convinced that our national association will fail of its highest opportunities and fall short of its best mission if it restricts itself to the narrow path of purely professional questions and withholds its interest and sympathy and its moral support from the great, urgent, throbbing, pressing social claims of our day and generation. Another is that I suspect many of you, absorbed in your

patients and your direct duties, are unaware of how rapidly this once revolutionary proposition is becoming a reality, or of how soon you may be called upon to respond to its actual presence in your midst.
Let us go over these reasons with a little more detail.

OUR GENERAL INDIFFERENCE

Of old the nursing sisters of the religious orders, closely confined in shackles of mental subjugation and social renunciation, consciously withdrew from all participation in things of the world, had no idea of preventive or constructive reforms, held no radical hopes of remaking the social order about them, but gave their lives to an unquestioning service of reparative and ameliorative devotion. If their paths were strewn with the wrecks of social justice they patiently and untiringly bound up the wounds and nursed the victims without a protest. If their hearts ever broke under the weight of preventable misery amidst which their lot was cast, they broke in silence. We have cast off their shackles, because we refuse to be cut off from the world about us. We have declared our principles to arise from another basis than theirs. We belong to an age which rejects the theory that misery and sickness are unpreventable,—which is learning to place prevention before amelioration, which is responding to the thrill of the discovery that the human race, as well as raw material, is capable of construction, of indefinite development and improvement; that human society can be voluntarily and consciously built into nobler and fairer forms than those of the past. If now, having secured the freedom which was denied to the sister of the religious orders, we shirk its responsibilities and ignore its duties, then we deliberately clothe ourselves again in her narrow-mindedness but without her holy zeal and self-consecration. Are we to choose for ourselves only the personal advantages of a greater freedom and to neglect the claims it makes upon our intelligence and our unselfishness? Those of you who are already keen and open-minded on this subject will bear me witness in reminding the indifferent ones of the story of the foolish virgins who were not ready when the call came. Women who are indifferent to the movement for political emancipation are often amazed when they are confronted with the facts of the actual advance of this social change.

As the modern nursing movement is emphatically an outcome of the original and general woman movement and as nurses are no longer a dull, uneducated class, but an intelligent army of workers, capable of continuous progress, and fitted to comprehend the idea of social responsibility, it would be a great pity for them to allow one of the most remarkable movements of the day to go on under their eyes without comprehending it. In the belief that such inattention actually exists in a large measure, I think it timely to present the following resume of the gradual extension of political equality to women up to the present time. It is a set of data sent by Miss Alice Stone Blackwell, one of the Editors of the Women's Journal, to the New York Evening Post:

"Seventy years ago women could not vote anywhere, except to a very limited extent in Sweden and a few other places in the Old World.

In 1838, Kentucky gave school suffrage to widows with children of school age. In 1850 Ontario gave it to women both married and single. In 1861 Kansas gave it to all women. Sweden gave women municipal suffrage in 1862, and New South Wales in 1867. In 1869 England gave municipal suffrage to single women and widows. Victoria gave it to women both married and single, and Wyoming gave municipal suffrage to all women. In 1871, West Australia gave municipal suffrage to women. School suffrage was granted in 1875 by Michigan and Minnesota, in 1876 by Colorado, in 1877 by New Zealand, in 1878 by New Hampshire and Oregon, in 1879 by Massachusetts, in 1880 by New York and Vermont. [In 1879, when the school suffrage was given to the women of Massachusetts, one of the members of the State Senate said, 'If we make this innovation, we shall destroy the race, which will be blasted by Almighty God.' I leave it to your common sense to decide how nearly right he was.] In 1880 South Australia gave municipal suffrage to women.

In 1881, municipal suffrage was extended to the single women and widows of Scotland, and Iceland gave single women and widows the right to vote for parish councils, district boards and vestries.

Nebraska gave women school suffrage in 1883. Municipal suffrage was given by Ontario and Tasmania in 1884, and by New Zealand and New Brunswick in 1886.

In 1887 municipal suffrage was granted in Kansas, Nova Scotia and Manitoba, and school suffrage in North and South Dakota, Montana, Arizona and New Jersey. In the same year Montana gave tax-paying women the right to vote upon all questions submitted to the taxpayers.

In 1888 England gave women county suffrage, and British Columbia and the Northwest Territory gave them municipal suffrage. In 1889 county suffrage was given to the women of Scotland, and municipal suffrage to single women and widows in the Province of Quebec. In 1891 school suffrage was granted in Illinois.

In 1893 school suffrage was granted in Connecticut, and full suffrage in Colorado and New Zealand. In 1894 school suffrage was granted in Ohio, bond suffrage in Iowa, church suffrage in Denmark, and parish and district suffrage in England to women both married and single. In 1895 full suffrage was granted in South Australia to women both married and single, and the right to vote for councillors to the women of Denmark. In 1896 full suffrage was granted in Utah and Idaho.

In 1897 Norway gave women a vote on certain church matters.

In 1898 the women of Iceland were given the right to vote for all officers except members of Parliament; Minnesota gave women the right to vote for

898 Report of the Tenth Annual Convention

library trustees; Delaware gave school suffrage to tax-paying women. France gave women engaged in commerce the right to vote for judges of the tribunals of commerce, and Louisiana gave tax-paying women the right to vote upon all questions submitted to the tax-payers. In 1900 Wisconsin gave women school suffrage and West Australia granted full parliamentary suffrage to women, both married and single.

In 1901 New York gave tax-paying women in all towns and villages of the state the right to vote on questions of local taxation. Norway gave women municipal suffrage, and the Kansas Legislature voted down almost unanimously, and 'amid a ripple of amusement,' a proposal to repeal municipal woman suffrage.

In 1902 full national suffrage was granted to all the women of federated Australia; state suffrage to the women of New South Wales, and Iceland made single women and widows eligible to all the offices for which they could vote, *i.e.*, as members of parish and town councils, district boards and vestries.

In 1903 bond suffrage was granted to the women of Queensland, and municipal suffrage to the women of Natal, South Africa.

In 1906 Finland gave women full national suffrage, and made them eligible to all offices, from members of Parliament down.

Within the last few weeks Finland has elected nineteen women to its Parliament."

This is the first instance in the history of the world of women being sent as members of a national legislature. Then, all of you who read the papers carefully, are aware how near the women of Great Britain came in the present session to obtaining the parliamentary franchise;— so near, indeed, that it was only snatched from them by a trick as base as it was desperate. But time does not permit me now to go into that discussion. What I want to make my main point is to insist upon the fast-coming change portended by all the signs of the times, and to ask: are we ready for it? What is to be our attitude toward full citizenship? Shall we be an intelligent and enlightened body of citizens, or an inert mass of indifference? Already our members in four western states enjoy political equality. How do they regard it? Do they realize their duties in this respect? Then, many of our members must live in communities where women have school suffrage. Do they exercise it? Let us now come to the position of our National Association on this subject, embracing as it does, let me repeat, the whole field of self-supporting industry and of education to prepare men and women for that industry. What I feel strongly is that our National Association might and should rise to a broader and more general consideration of large, general subjects than it has heretofore done, or than our local bodies, perhaps, have time to do, though these also, I believe, might well broaden the scope of their interests.

Our local bodies must, however, always carry many details of our professional lives. They must concern themselves with many practical questions, law-making, registration, sick benefit funds, the ethical standards of members and a thousand Martha-like cares. I would like to see our national body leave all smaller concerns to the local societies and consciously make itself a moral force on all the great social questions of the day. Of old we have at times discussed in our national and state meetings, such trivial difficulties as uniforms, perplexities arising from personal preferences of patients for one nurse over another. But now the day has come when we might here decide on our place, our share, and our policy toward the great social claims of education and educational reforms,—industry and the industrial situation—especially as it relates to women—child-labor, its iniquities and dangers (no question more than this has a direct bearing on the public health or the spread of tuberculosis, in which we are taking an active prophylactic part, and none is more sinister in its influence on education); prostitution and the white slave traffic with its trail of disease and death, and the recent movement to teach sexual hygiene, to inculcate a single moral standard, and to combat venereal disease of which we make so melancholy an acquaintance—not only in the wards of city hospitals but even among our private patients; this, one of the newest reform and educational movements, proves perhaps more strikingly than any other that a new conception of human society has arisen and that a new ideal is to be pursued for the future. I am far from thinking that many of us individually can take any active or direct part in extending these various propaganda, but to all of such movements we could give at least intelligent sympathy and moral support—perhaps occasionally some useful service—certainly often our mite in money, and so closely are all the threads of modern life intertwined that it is a question how long we may as an organized society withhold our interest from these subjects and yet demand the interest and the respect of society as a whole for ourselves and our individual problems. I would like to hear these great social questions discussed in our meetings. I would like to have our journals not afraid to mention the words political equality for women. I would like to see our local groups give more time to a consideration of their relation to other bodies of workers, for it has been said by a wise person that those who only know their own specialty do not even know that one. Consider, for instance, for a moment, the relation of our own educational problem to the present conditions of industrial life. We are absorbed in the effort to establish and maintain a sound preliminary education for women desiring to become nurses. But as, in the final event, most women who become nurses will do so because they wish to support themselves, we must observe what conditions are affecting the great mass of self-supporting women. We then find that the industrial tide is sweeping thousands of young women into occupations at younger and ever younger age, ever less and less well prepared for their occupations by education, training, and discipline, and we then, observing farther, find armies of children, literally armies, for there are nearly two million, underbidding these young women and older children in self-supporting occupations, losing their school time, destroying their physique and preparing a racial deterioration. These millions of children are dragging down the general standards of education and training all over the country wherever they are—and will not many of them in the future lower the standards of coming generations of nurses? For no higher education can remain sound and stable unless it is based on adequate primary instruction and effective manual training. Such by-paths link our destiny with that of every other worker.

To those who are keenly interested in movement for political equality it is very significant to note the gradual change in the tone of the press, and to see such publications as Harper's Weekly, and the North American Review, come out openly in advocacy of the political enfranchisement of women. The fact is that modern industrial society is creating a set of conditions which can only be met and properly handled by legally giving women the same place in public affairs which has been her traditional place in the home, for now the home is reaching out into every ramification of public life. For a general and clear statement of this idea nothing is better than a pamphlet written by Miss Jane Addams, called "The Modern City and the Municipal Franchise for Women." It explains the altered conception of the modern city, compared with that of the mediæval one. The problems of the modern city are almost entirely housekeeping questions on a vast scale. The cleanliness and healthfulness of the city must be simply extensions of the cleanliness and healthfulness of the home; the care of children needs now to be extended to the public school, to the factory, to the shop,— even to the courts, and to the prisons. The care of the young must be extended to the street, to the temptations put in their way by franchise-holding men; to the badhouses, to the saloons, again to the courts, to the jails, to the halls where laws are framed. The health and happiness of the home and the vigor of the mother of future generations must be protected in factories, in sweat-shops, in caravansery launderies, in vast unhygienic business establishments,—four snug walls no longer bound the domain of the home. These responsibilities do not belong to men alone nor can these conditions longer be met and adjusted with that organ of self-expression, the ballot. I have been much impressed lately by what I have seen of enlightened women, going disfranchised, to legislative assemblies to struggle, handicapped, in defence of the children in industry against men, strong in entrenched forts of governmental rule and armed with their ballots. It is a distressing and a pitiable sight. This was in my own state which has a bad record in this respect. In the western free states, the women secure, without a tithe of the nerve-rack, better conditions of labor and of education for their children than those of eastern states can secure by their influence. And I have been intent on the struggle of the women teachers in New York State for the justice of equal payment. The only states in the union where women teachers are paid the same as men are the four free states of the west. So far, in our own legislation, we have been fairly successful, but let me close with this prophecy: Until we possess the ballot we shall not know when we may get up in the morning to find that all we had gained has been taken from us.

THE PRESIDENT.—The paper is open for discussion.

MISS DAVIS.—Madam president, I have been asked to lead the discussion on this paper. I had not the remotest idea of the trend of it, but I am sure that many thinking people believe in giving the ballot to women. We all believe that were the franchise granted to women, the administration of existing laws would be much more effective, and the making of new laws would be much more effective, more exact, and much more humane; for the laws that already exist are good laws but their administration is not always along the lines of humanity. We are striving in a small way to gain legislation in our profession, and to take hold of this question might injure us, and probably would. I do not think Miss Dock means that; I think she means we should discuss such questions and inform ourselves along such lines, and, as we are all well-disciplined, high-thinking women, when the time comes to act we shall know how to make laws and how to have them properly administered. I would like to hear from some of the states that have the franchise, how much more they are able to do along these lines than we are in states that have not the franchise for women.

MISS BOYD.—Madam president, personally I do not believe in women having the franchise. I have been west for thirteen years; I went to Colorado when women first obtained the right to vote. It was intensely interesting to me because I came from New York where everything is conservative, and I attended all the meetings and I was very sorry I had not a chance to cast my ballot. In the course of time I became a citizen and I did vote, and then I became interested in nursing work; now I believe it is a duty, and as long as the privilege is given to the women of that state they should exercise that privilege and cast their ballots. The last election we had there was probably the best that Colorado has had. Before that the better class of women left the ballot to the women in the lower half of the town—I am speaking of Denver specially—and they carried things their own way which was not the best way for the community. This last time, by a new election law whereby the voters are registered in their homes, the bad registration lists were restricted, and the better class of women came out and cast their ballots, and we had a much better and cleaner election. I am not able to answer Miss Davis' question. Women have been in the legislature, but it seems to me that when you go into politics, there are a great many things you have to take up if you go into it fully, and we loose a little something as women, I cannot help feeling that. I think the making of citizenship comes before a person is ten years old, I don't think it comes after twenty-one; and I think that Judge Lindsey in his work among the children and people of Denver is doing much more for citizenship than all the women votes of Colorado.

MISS DOCK.—How has Judge Lindsey been able to hold his position? The women of Colorado have kept him in office against the combined efforts of corruption in that state. It is the women of Colorado who have made it possible for Judge Lindsey to save their children.

MRS. ROBB.—Madam president, I would like to have a moment to speak on an urgent social claim that has been called to my attention by being asked in my home city to give lectures on hygiene to our school children, by reading two articles in THE AMERICAN JOURNAL OF NURSING, and by having my attention called first to the fact that at the last June meeting of the Medical Association of America there was a symposium of papers presented by a doctor there upon what he called the two great social evils of the present time, the two plagues of the present century; he termed them the white plague and the black plague, and said that we must turn our attention to doing something more than we have been doing to wipe them out of existence. Then THE AMERICAN JOURNAL OF NURSING called your attention to that symposium of papers. The JOURNAL also gave us articles on what it called Venereal Prophylaxis. I think if the JOURNAL never gave us anything but those articles, it is worth everything we have done for it. I want to beg you, when you go back home, to take those numbers and read those articles over carefully once more, and then consider what claim there is upon us as professional women to assist the doctors in stamping out these two plagues in this country. One is tuberculosis and the other is venereal diseases. I was very strongly impressed, and I thought it my duty this last winter, though I have very many matters to occupy me, to speak to the children on hygiene; I commenced with anatomy and physiology, and it was most impressive to me to see how the little eyes and ears opened for instruction about the human body, to know something about themselves and to be told it in such a way that they could take it in and apply it practically in every-day life.

I gave another course of lectures on hygiene to a class of women preparing for work as kindergarteners. Before giving the lectures, I asked those of the students who had had instruction in anatomy and physiology to stand up, so that I might know how intelligently they would be able to receive my remarks on hygiene. Less than one-third of the women stood up, and they were all high school graduates.

Now it seems to me that there are two bodies who are distinctly educators, the teachers of our country and ourselves, and it seems to me that our special line of education, as we know how important it is to advance preventive medicine, is to take just this one particular line of work for our own in our local associations, to create first a public sentiment for teaching anatomy and physiology, not as it is attempted to be taught to-day in our public schools and high schools and private schools, to boys and girls together, but as it ought to be taught, practically, and with demonstrations, so that the pupils will be able to apply it, for them to be taught it until they become grown young men and women, and do away with this ignorance, this great mystery, of the human body as the general public considers it, make them realize what their bodies are, and the uses and abuses of them; and I think we will have less need to nurse those two great diseases.

I would just like to make this suggestion. Our president in her opening address touched upon our duties from an educational standpoint, and I felt, after Miss Dock's paper, that perhaps we ought not to go away to our homes in distant states without a definite line to work upon. It seems to me that public school teachers, generally speaking, are not in the position to teach anatomy and physiology that trained nurses are in. I know one woman who came to me in connection with her sister who had to have an operation; she said, "I don't know anything about that because I don't know anything about the human body." Another woman of fifty to whom a nurse was giving massage, said, "What are muscles?" I could tell you many things about the deplorable ignorance of women about the abuses of the human body, and these are the things we are fighting. The great problems we have to meet are results, as we know, of ignorance on that one subject. We would not have so many patients in the hospitals, we would not need so many hospitals, if people knew more about the human body. So don't you think it possible for us to create a sentiment in our different towns upon the necessity of teaching children, practically and intelligently, those subjects of anatomy and physiology, and then to apply the rules of hygiene? Do you not think we should create teachers for that purpose? It is not necessary that one woman should be appointed to every school, but if we had one good woman for the schools of a city, she could go from one school to another and teach so that every child in the city would have that instruction. You have taken a great step towards that in your liberal contribution to the Hospital Economics course; that was originally created especially for women who wished to become hospital superintendents, but I have been going there every year to give my share toward the teaching and I have been meeting women coming back for the second year. There are three or four of them who have not any intention of ever becoming superintendents of training-schools, but they are taking special courses in anatomy, physiology and psychology and are being taught how to teach, how to impart that knowledge to others. They are splendid women, and my eyes were opened to the possibility of using these women taking that special training for these special lines in our training-schools, it will help us tremendously; and now comes another opening for them if we can introduce them into our public schools and private schools for boys and girls and give them the right knowledge of how to care for the human body, how to use it and how to reverence it, so that they will not have these diseases.

THE PRESIDENT.—It seems a most opportune moment to take up the suggestion made by our board of directors, that we have a Committee on Public Health in this Association. If that is your pleasure, a motion to appoint such a committee will be in order before we adjourn to-day.

Miss McMillan.—I move that the president appoint a Committee on Public Health.

The motion was seconded and carried.

The President.—I do not feel that I can appoint that very important committee on the spur of the moment, but it will be appointed at the directors' meeting and the announcement made. Are there any other topics to discuss?

Miss Davis.—Madam president, I have here an appeal to the nurses of America, coming from a number of superintendents of training-schools, calling the attention of the nurses to the proposition of a certain Insurance Company, which has arranged special rates for nurses.

It has been partially investigated, and found to be a good investment, and a reasonably safe proposition. I have been asked to put this before the society, but as I know so very little about it, I think it had better be investigated or discussed, or something done to it by this assembly.

Miss DeWitt.—This is such an important matter, and it is so hard for a large body to investigate the details of a business proposition like this, that I move it be referred to the board of directors for investigation.

The motion was duly seconded and adopted.

Miss McIsaac.—Madam president, I would like to ask that a committee be appointed during the coming year for the consideration of the subject of an annuity fund, or something of that sort, for nurses. I do not know enough about the phraseology of matters of that kind to put it properly, but I move that a committee be appointed to look into that matter in conjunction with the superintendents' society, and the state societies, to see if we cannot among ourselves do something of the same nature that the insurance companies do.

The President.—Do you want this committee appointed by the directors?

Miss McIsaac.—By the Chair.

Miss Jamme.—Would it take too long a time to have some statement from Miss Dock as to what the European nurses are doing?

Miss Dock.—Germany has state insurance for all working people, which is very different from any other country; we can't get that. It is a very respectable thing because the worker and employer contribute, and the state adds a tax. The taxes are not large, but they are something, and the Nurses' Association there insists on all the members joining the Government insurance.

The strong point about the Government insurance is that you do not have to pass a physical examination.

The German Nurses' Association says to a member, "We want you to do all you can for your own self help, and after that the organization will help you, but if you neglect the means of helping yourself, which are open to you, then you must not expect other people to assist you."

That works very well. The German organizations have an emergency fund. The English nurses have not any good system whatever; it has been in the past the custom of certain hospitals and certain institutions to pay the nurses a certain sum, after a certain length of time; that is very nice, but of course it is very limited. They have there what I consider the most objectionable system of insurance existing in any country, the Royal Pension Fund, gotten up by Mr. Burdette, which is made by some hospitals obligatory upon its pupils, which I think is altogether odious, objectionable, impertinent and tyrannous. It is simply an insurance. I have never been able to find that its benefits are in any way better than those offered by the insurance companies, not as favorable as those offered by the German insurance companies, which are perfectly business-like. And then there has always been connected with the British Pension Fund a most objectionable flavor of patronage. The names of the nurses who join it are published, and there has always been a most objectionable flavor of patronage, condescension, and almost charity.

Of the independent organized nurses, ninety-nine out of a hundred, I think, do not belong to it, and they have no such sick benefit funds as we have, nothing organized on a general scale.

MISS GREENTHAL.—Madam president, I would like to say that the Mount Sinai Association is at present founding a Pension Fund in connection with our alumnæ association, and trying to have it incorporated. Just now we have had some trouble in that respect on account of the insurance laws, but we hope to succeed.

The motion to appoint a committee to look into the insurance subject was duly seconded and adopted, and the president appointed on the committee, Miss M. E. P. Davis, Miss Anna C. Jamme, and Miss M. L. Wyche.

"The London Meeting of the International
 Council and Congress of Nurses"

     Dock's account of the London meeting of the
International Council of Nurses in 1909 (American
Journal of Nursing 10 [October 1909]: 15-21) conveys
some idea of the excitement and enthusiasm that
infused these gatherings. Such person-to-person
contacts in this and other organizations at the
time encouraged many to harbor dreams of permanent
friendship among nations, dreams that would be
rudely shattered in 1914 with the outbreak of the
Great War.

THE LONDON MEETING OF THE INTERNATIONAL COUNCIL AND CONGRESS OF NURSES

By LAVINIA L. DOCK, R.N.

Honorary Secretary International Council of Nurses

THE OFFICIAL DAY.—Each assemblage of nurses, of an international character, has been bigger, more deeply enthusiastic, more inspiring than the last. So the meetings of the London Quinquennial have been not only more remarkable than any others for intense interest and for their cosmopolitan character, but also for the powerful energy of impulse felt by all present, which was expressed in ways that will bring far-reaching results.

First, who was there? Seventeen countries were represented by delegates, fraternal delegates, or visitors, and eight or nine languages were heard, though English was spoken throughout on the platform. Official delegates present were: Mrs. Bedford Fenwick, president of the National Council of Trained Nurses of Great Britain and Ireland, and four delegates from that body who were, Miss Rogers, matron of the Leicester Infirmary, Miss Lamont, superintendent of the Irish branch of the Queen Victoria Jubilee Institute, Miss Burleigh, superintendent of the Royal Hospital for Sick Children, Edinburgh, and Miss Burr, secretary of the League of St. John's House Nurses. Miss Goodrich, R.N., president, and Mrs. Robb, Miss Delano, R.N., Miss Maxwell, R.N., and Miss Cadmus, R.N., delegates of the American Federation of Nurses. Sister Agnes Karll, R.N., president, and Sisters Erna Nagel, R.N., recently from the International Hospital, Palermo, Italy; Marthe Franke, R.N., matron of the Children's Seashore Sanatorium, Norderney; Hedwig Schmidts, R.N., assistant matron, City Hospital, Charlottenburg, and Hanna Miller, R.N., superintendent of the City Hospital, Rheydt, sent by the German Nurses' Association. Miss Tilanus, president of the Holland Nurses' Association, and Miss van Lanschot Hubrecht, the secretary of the same, Miss Verbeck, district nurse in the municipal medical service, Amsterdam; Miss van Haeften, the first appointed public school nurse in Holland; and Miss Meyboom, matron of one of the city hospitals, Rotterdam, as delegates from Holland. Baroness Mannerheim, matron of the Surgical Hospital, Helsingfors, and president of the Association of Nurses of Finland, with Miss Koreneff, matron of the Maria Hospital, Helsingfors; Miss Nylander, superintendent of the Preliminary Training School of the

Helsingfors Surgical Hospital; Miss Bergstrom, hospital Sister, and Mrs. Lackstrom, editor of *Epione,* the journal of the Finnish nurses, delegates. Mrs. Tscherning, president of the Danish Council of Nurses, with the four Danish delegates, Miss Hellfach, superintending nurse in the Kommune Hospital, Copenhagen; Mrs. Koch, recently head nurse in the Presbyterian Hospital, New York City, now living in Denmark; Miss Hjorth, Sister in the Royal Frederiks Hospital, Copenhagen, and Miss Andersen, Sister in the Qresunds Hospital, Copenhagen. Miss Snively, president of the Canadian National Association of Trained Nurses, with the Canadian delegates, Miss Brent, superintendent of the Hospital for Sick Children, Toronto; Miss Scott, superintendent of the Training School, Grace Hospital, Toronto; Miss Baikie, president of the Montreal branch, and Miss Tedford, head nurse in the General Hospital, Montreal. Such a delegation has never yet been seen in the history of nursing.

Other members present with votes were seven officers and councillors of the International, and two honorary vice-presidents, namely, Miss Breay, treasurer, and Miss Dock, secretary, and Miss Stewart, matron of St. Bartholomew's Hospital; Miss Cureton, Miss Knight, matron of the General Hospital, Nottingham; Miss Mollett, matron of the Royal South Hants and Southampton Hospital, and Miss Huxley, past president of the Irish Nurses' Association (and niece of the great Huxley), councillors, Dr. Anna Hamilton, France, and Miss Turton, Italy, honorary vice-presidents.

Furthermore came the fraternal delegates, having no votes, but coming to show good-will and interest. From Australia five, Miss Robson, Miss Blomfield, Miss Ragg, Miss Peyton Jones, and Miss Laurence, as well as several visitors from Australia; from Cuba three, Miss Hibbard, whose work is so well known and who is now directing tuberculosis work in Havana, Miss Nuñez, inspector-general of schools for nurses under the Cuban government, and president of the Cuban Nurses' Association, and Miss Monteagudo, superintendent of the Municipal Sanitary Service, Havana. These fraternal delegates were sent by the government Department of Health and Charities. All their expenses were paid, and they brought most kind and cordial letters from the head of the department, Dr. Duque, whose interest in the wider education of his nurses is a gratifying thing and an example to be followed.

Belgium sent prominent fraternal delegates, several of whom came directly from the Belgian government and several from the Federation of Secular Nursing Schools. Miss Cavell, superintendent of the training school in Brussels, read the report, and Dr. Ley, the advanced physician who came from Paris, was again present, while several nurses completed the party.

France sent a remarkable body of fraternal delegates, representing all the modern progressive groups in that country. Besides Dr. Hamilton, Miss Elston, Dr. Lande, and Mme. Kriegk came from Bordeaux, with Mlle. Siegrist, one of their graduates now in charge of a maternity school, Mlle. Irasque, and Mlle. Bos, assistant and pupil from the Tondu; Mlle. Luigi, the young superintendent of hospital and training school at Béziers and president of the French Society of Training School Superintendents, came also, while the French Minister of War appointed Mlle. Roullet to represent army nurses.

From Paris came Mme. Jacques, the attractive and gracious matron of the new training school in Paris, with a group of her pupils; M. André Mesureur and the new director of the Salpêtrière, representing the governmental department of Hospitals and Charities of Paris; Mlle. Chaptal and Mme. Alphen-Salvador, representing the private nursing schools; and ladies representing the French Red Cross Society.

Fraternal delegates came from Holland representing the conservative party.

Japan, through the kind personal interest of our old friend Miss Suwo, and of Prince Matsukata, president of the Red Cross Society of Japan, sent a most engaging little fraternal delegate in the person of Miss Take Hagiwara, who has served through three wars and received medals from France and Japan. She attended all the sessions most regularly, brought a splendid paper from Japan, and was quite one of the lions.

Sweden sent a very notable group of fraternal delegates, forty in all, headed by Miss Tamm and representing all the important hospitals, training schools, and the nursing journal of that country. They came under the direct auspices of the Dowager Queen of Sweden, who takes an active interest in nursing matters, and who is to receive full accounts of all the movements now under way in the nursing world.

Switzerland also sent a fraternal delegate from the pioneer school La Source.

New Zealand sent Miss Maude and Miss Palmer, while nurses came as visitors from Norway, Ireland, Scotland, and from all the countries already mentioned. Germany sent forty in all, every one registered under the imperial registration Act; Denmark sent forty-three all told; Canada some fifteen or more beside the delegates; American nurses who attended the meetings numbered about twenty-four in addition to the delegates; and the English nurses in attendance cannot well be estimated.

Among the Americans were Miss Packard and Miss Martin, Baltimore; Miss Le Van, Miss Giberson, and Miss Krause, Philadelphia; Miss Ehrlicher and Miss Pindell, Superintendents' Society; Miss Pearson, now in Cuba, while the thoroughly representative character of the American delegation was completed in an unexpected and gratifying manner by the appearance, at the last moment, of the Editor-in-Chief of the AMERICAN JOURNAL OF NURSING, Miss Sophia F. Palmer.

Church House Hall, holding fifteen hundred persons, was filled on Monday; about six hundred tickets were issued to the large receptions, and four hundred and fourteen nurses, mostly foreigners, went to Windsor. This will give an idea of numbers.

A glorious atmosphere of expectant enthusiasm was felt in the beautiful hall of the Church House on Monday, the opening and official day. The organ accompanied the entrance of our hundreds of visitors, and the platform and body of the hall were packed as Mrs. Fenwick arose, in her capacity as honorary president, to open the meeting. She expressed the one regret at the absence of Miss McGahey, the president, and then, in an eloquent address, gave the watchword for the coming period—" Life." The reports from the three federated countries were read, and then Miss Goodrich, on behalf of the American Federation of Nurses, extended to Mrs. Fenwick and Miss Isla Stewart the invitation unanimously given by that body in Minneapolis to accept honorary membership in its midst. They accepted with pleasure, and both invitation and acceptance were accompanied by bouquets of roses. The four councils of Holland, Finland, Denmark, and Canada were then affiliated. This was a beautiful and impressive ceremony. As each incoming president in turn read her report she was greeted by a speech of welcome and a beautiful bouquet, and the national anthem of her country was played on the organ. All present rose to each anthem, while many voices took up the strains of beloved patriotic airs. Enthusiasm was intense as these splendid leaders of nursing progress responded individually to the welcome given them.

Officers for the next period were then elected: Sister Agnes Karll as the next president, while Miss Breay and Miss Dock were re-elected. Sister Agnes's first words were a greeting to Miss Nightingale, the revered woman and pioneer.

The amendments to the constitution were quickly despatched. The number of delegates is to remain as now, four from each country, but the fees were reduced. The time between regular meetings was altered from five to three years. The next meeting will take place in 1912, and in Cologne, as Sister Agnes believes that it will help German progress.

The purpose of the International is first of all to be helpful and to go where it can give aid and stimulus.

The resolutions next came up. The first, on registration, was passed unanimously. It was put by Mrs. Robb and seconded by Mrs. Kock. A dramatic incident then occurred. Up rose Mr. Sydney Holland, time-worn enemy of registration and upholder of the system of sending undergraduates to private duty. Asking when he could be heard in opposition, he stated that the meeting was not representative. Some nurses hissed, and Miss Dock asked why he then thought it worth while to come before it with his views. Excitement was quelled by the chair who declared that full opportunity for discussion would be given next day. The enemy, followed by a henchman, then retreated in good order. The second resolution, on the rights of citizenship, was then put by Miss Hubrecht, and seconded by the Baroness Mannerheim, who told of what the women of Finland were doing with the ballot. Mrs. Millicent G. Fawcett, one of England's women prominent in higher education, had brought greetings and spoken on citizenship before the resolution was put. No dissent was expressed. Forty-two voting members being present, it was carried by a vote of thirty-eight in the affirmative. Two members voted in the negative, two refrained from voting, and two were absent. Reports were then read from countries not affiliated. Enthusiasm arose afresh for the foreign fraternal delegates on the platform, and all the reports were of great interest.

The meeting came to an end with profound emotions of joy and uplift, and all adjourned to the Gaiety Restaurant where several hundred were entertained at luncheon, amidst flowers, music, and jollity, by Mrs. Fenwick and a group of the English nurses. In all its fulness of serious interest, picturesque ceremonial, and unity of feeling this was a day the like of which we have never had.

THE CONGRESS.—The remaining four days were given to open congress meetings, of most varied interest, excellent papers, and thronged attendance. The first session in Caxton Hall was devoted to Education and Registration. Dr. Beard's paper, presented at Minneapolis, had a place here and is regarded as most important and valuable by the English leaders. Another dramatic scene occurred when Mr. Sydney Holland reappeared, armed with a very long, dull, and unconvincing brief against registration. Before beginning it he offered gross personal discourtesies to our English hostesses by launching into belittling remarks as to the relative sizes of their training schools and hospitals, and was called to order to speak to the subject under discussion. Again he descended to personalities, and meanly libelled an English nurse present, who promptly came to the platform and exposed his " inaccuracies." Great sensation reigned. Cries of " shame," " out of order," " unfair," were heard, and it was with difficulty the chairman could secure him a hearing. After all he never came to any point, over-ran his time, and had to be closed off by the bell. As an opponent he showed himself not an honorable enemy, but a mean one, and he carried with him from the hall the general contempt of those present who understood the question. It was a perfect demonstration of what the progressive party in England have had to battle against during the past twenty years.

Deeply interesting sessions were held on " Private Duty," " School Nursing," and " The Nurse as Citizen." In the latter many of the new preventive lines of work were brought out. " The Relations of Nursing and Medicine" and the " Care of the Insane " elicited much interest. Dr. Russell's paper, given at Minneapolis, was read again here. The " Nurse as Patriot " gave the army nursing service a hearing. The session on " Morality and Health" was a terribly earnest one, and " Mission Nursing " closed the most successful and inspiring congress that we have ever held.

SOCIAL FUNCTIONS.—The extent and beauty of the social entertainments, the unbounded hospitality shown us, and the perfect arrangements and foresight of the British nurses are quite indescribable. Only those few individuals who came late or unannounced had the smallest uncertainty. Weeks ago all the tickets and invitation cards, six or eight each, were addressed to every foreign visitor who was known to be coming. The reception given by Miss Isla Stewart in the Great Hall of St. Bartholomew's Hospital was perhaps the most unique and never-to-be-forgotten evening. Another remarkable one was the banquet, where Lord Ampthill, champion of registration and typical example of the chivalrous English gentleman, presided. The receptions given by Mrs. Whitelaw Reid at Dorchester House and the Lord Mayor and Lady Mayoress at the Mansion House were both beautiful. The " conversazione " at the charming Doré gallery and the " At Home " of the *British Journal of Nursing* in Caxton Hall, the tea at the Irish Village at the Exhibition at Shepherd's Bush, with Irish songs and dances, potato cakes, scones, strawberries, and tea; the reception at St. John's House, the Nurses' Lodge, and, finally, the visit to Windsor, made a week of varied, brilliant, and lovely impressions. The king himself took a special interest in the visit to Windsor, permitting us to see galleries and gardens not shown to tourists, and allowing the loyal Canadians to lay a wreath on the tomb of Queen Victoria.

WORK OUTLINED BY THE CONGRESS.—As outcome of the papers and discussions two important lines of work are to be undertaken. One, at the suggestion of Mrs. Robb, will be a standing international committee on education to confer and work toward agreement of the basic requirements in the training of nurses. The other, the appointment of a national committee in each country to work up the propaganda against venereal disease. The congress also passed a resolution recommending courses of instruction for warders and wardresses in prisons.

REPORTS OF THE CONGRESS.—The reports given weekly by the *British Journal of Nursing* have been very remarkable, and the fulness, detail, and variety as well as accuracy of this journal's account of the whole meeting constitute a wonderful journalistic feat. The *International* will publish an official report, cost 25 cents (one shilling), but this will not contain the four days' congress papers. These will appear from time to time in the British and American journals. The report may be ordered, prepaid, from 2131 Oxford Street, London, W.

The various groups of nurses who had planned and arranged the exhibits deserve the highest praise for the remarkably interesting displays made and for the celerity with which they were all put into place. The district nursing exhibit filled a whole room and was remarkably well done. Every possible sort of device, contrivance, and invention that the ingenuity of nurse or patient could devise was there, and it seems a pity that this most instructive exhibit could not be made a permanent or a travelling one, for nothing quite like it has ever been seen before. The organizers of this section were Lady Hermione Blackwood, Queen's nurse, Miss du Sautoy, a county superintendent of the Queen's nurses, and Miss Eden, who gave great thought and ability to their task. The district nursing exhibit received and well merited the first prize.

St. John's House exhibit, illustrating maternity work and the collection organized by the Leicester Infirmary Nurses' League, demonstrating the care of the eye, ear, nose, and throat were admirably done, as also the Irish exhibit, containing many excellent inventions. The school nurses' exhibit, the London Missionary School of Medicine exhibit, the mortuary exhibit arranged by Miss Greenstreet, and the St. Bartholomew's League exhibit containing much of historical interest were all noteworthy. From abroad came many excellent exhibits, the German Nurses' Association sending a remarkable collection of over fifty dolls in various uniforms. There were also beautiful collections of badges, etc. Our space does not permit us sufficient detail, and we refer our readers to the issues of July 17 and July 24 of the *British Journal of Nursing*.

Hygiene and Morality

Many nurses, including Lavinia Dock, took part in the public campaign against tuberculosis in the early 1900s, but Dock was one of the few women who joined another, more daring campaign, against venereal disease. Even more daring was publishing a book on the subject, in which she discussed not only VD but prostitution and sexuality as well. Dock's Hygiene and Morality is of historical interest for its delineation of Progressive reform attitudes toward these subjects, then only beginning to be openly talked about.

The book's title states its message. Social hygiene was the euphemism for VD prevention. Morality meant the means: abolition of prostitution. The discovery of salvarsan, the first effective treatment for syphilis, had been announced in 1910, but Dock, and many physicians, had little enthusiasm for therapy, believing that without fear of infection as a deterrent, "animal passions" might run riot.

Prostitution was becoming a reform target in many cities. Jane Addams and other settlement workers, who had discovered that prostitutes were not the "fallen women" of the popular stereotype, were prodding the public conscience. This generation of middle-class reformers, reared on Victorian fears of sexuality (note Dock's strictures on masturbation), envisioned a new, loftier sexual morality. A single standard would prevail. Abolition of prostitution would end the exploitation of women through what was widely assumed to be an organized "white slave traffic." Male sexuality would then be confined within marriage.

The Victorians had taught that women were passionless; now, Dock wrote, "our foremost medical teachers" emphasized that men suffered no loss of health by sexual restraint. In the new moral order, "[t]he generative act," representing "the noblest of human powers," would "only be performed in the sincerity of aspiration to bring a new being into the world."

Dock had embraced the popular science of eugenics, which further fanned Progressive hopes of improving the human race. To this end she added a plea for the mitigation of poverty and for political and legal equality for women. Her book had only a short life before the advent of World War I, followed by middle-class adoption of birth control and Freudian psychology, changed the climate of opinion and closed this chapter in the history of sexual ideology.

By Lavinia L. Dock

A TEXT-BOOK OF MATERIA MEDICA FOR NURSES. Fourth Edition, Revised and Enlarged. Cr. 8vo. Net, $1.50

HISTORY OF NURSING. The Evolution of the Methods of Care for the Sick from the Earliest Times to the Foundation of the First English and American Training Schools for Nurses. By LAVINIA L. DOCK, R.N., and M. ADELAIDE NUTTING, R.N. Two volumes, 8vo. Fully illustrated. Net, $5.00.

Hygiene and Morality

A Manual for Nurses and Others, Giving an Outline of the Medical, Social, and Legal Aspects of the Venereal Diseases

By

Lavinia L. Dock, R.N.

Graduate of Bellevue Hospital Training School, Resident Member of the Nurses' Settlement, New York, Secretary of the International Council of Nurses

G. P. Putnam's Sons
New York and London
The Knickerbocker Press
1910

Copyright, 1910
by
LAVINIA L. DOCK

The Knickerbocker Press, New York

PREFACE

THE plan of this manual has grown from the scope of a paper presented by the author to the International Congress of Nurses in London, in July, 1909, in which the chief purpose aimed at was the same as has been here followed, namely, to reiterate the social significance of the venereal diseases and the crusade upon which women should enter in regard to them. Therefore, though the book is meant primarily for the nursing profession with its many thousands of members, it has not been arranged simply as a text-book on diseases, and the author hopes it may be useful to many other women as well. The author's thanks are to be cordially expressed to Dr. Elizabeth Hurdon and Dr. Florence Sabin, both of the Johns Hopkins Medical School, for reading the text on the Venereal Diseases; to Dr. Caroline Hedger, member of the Chicago Society of Social Hygiene, who has read the whole text; to Dr. Louis I. Dublin of Brooklyn for information relating to industrial insurance, and to Miss Alice Henry of Hull House for notes on maternal subsidies.

LAVINIA L. DOCK, R. N.

The Nurses' Settlement
265 Henry St., New York.

CONTENTS

CHAPTER   PAGE

PART I.—THE VENEREAL DISEASES   1

I. SYPHILIS 3

II. GONORRHŒA AND CHANCROID . . 40

PART II.—PROSTITUTION   57

I. CONTROL AND REGULATION OF PROSTITUTION 59

II. THE WHITE SLAVE TRAFFIC . . . 104

PART III. THE PREVENTION OF VENEREAL DISEASE   127

I. UNDERLYING PRINCIPLES OF PREVENTION . 129

APPENDICES 171

INDEX 195

Part I. The Venereal Diseases

CHAPTER I

SYPHILIS

THE venereal diseases are, in the commonly accepted order of their gravity: Syphilis; Gonorrhœa; Chancroid. The first mentioned is, by many modern medical writers, classed by itself, as will be explained later. For a long period in medical history, these three were all believed to be manifestations of one and the same disease. This confusion of ideas continued until the identification of the specific causative germs brought definite understanding and gave a sound basis to theory.

HISTORICAL OUTLINE. Venereal diseases are of great, probably of unknown antiquity. Some writers say that gonorrhœa has always existed. Syphilis appears to accompany certain stages of civilisation, as at least some barbarous tribes are and have been free from it. It is known that it has been introduced into certain ones of such tribes by white men. This has recently occurred with decimating results in the case of the tribe of Baganzas in Central Africa.

Some medical historians affirm that syphilis was unknown in Europe before the discovery of America and that it was carried thence into Europe, having presumably had its source in the ancient civilisations of Central America. Prominent authorities hold · this view, while others, also prominent, maintain that it has existed for many more centuries in Europe but has been confused with leprosy. The controversy is one of no more than academic interest. What is historically certain is, that an epidemic of syphilis of frightful virulence raged in Europe at the end of the fifteenth century, constituting a veritable plague, and that it spread to all the countries and corners of the continent. Since then, it has been ever present in a less spectacular, sub-acute form as an endemic disease. Though now less noticeable, it is no less pestilential; perhaps indeed it is even more dangerous by reason of its concealment, as it is thus able to promote undiscovered that racial degeneration which has been pointed out as one of its chief activities.

CAUSE OF SYPHILIS. Syphilis is caused by a

Syphilis

micro-organism called the *Spirochæte pallida* of Schaudinn. This micro-organism, the specific and invariable cause of syphilis, has not long been known with certainty, though long before its actual demonstration medical specialists had suspected its existence. Metchnikoff records the work of Donné, a French microscopist, who, in 1837, tried to learn from his microscope the exact nature of the genito-urinary discharge in both men and women. But his efforts resulted in nothing definite. In his day the germ theory was nonexistent. After the work of Pasteur had given a new direction to medical and surgical study and had caused the doctrine of the action of microorganisms as the cause of infectious disease to be accepted, active search and research went on in laboratories all over the world, to discover the germs of this as well as of other diseases. But for twenty years or more the definite attempts made by Weigart, Lustgarten, Metchnikoff, and many others to find the cause of syphilis ended in failure. Finally a commission of experts was formed under the lead of Schulze, Professor of Zoölogy in the University of Berlin, and the investigation directed toward the discovery of the syphilitic virus was by him entrusted to Schaudinn and Hoffman, who, finally, were successful in their search, and in 1905 were able to demonstrate the micro-organism which is now generally accepted by the medical profession as the cause of syphilis.

SCHAUDINN'S DISCOVERY. It was shown that two varieties of *Spirilla* were to be found in normal and in diseased states of the genital organs. The first variety, called *Spirilla refringens*, may be existent in either state, and may be demonstrated in different pathological conditions, both non-syphilitic and syphilitic in character. The second variety, the *Spirilla pallida*, is only found in syphilis, not even in other venereal diseases unless syphilis is also present.

THE SPIROCHÆTE PALLIDA. The *Spirochæte pallida* is classed among the *Spirilla*. It is not yet definitely settled whether it belongs to the bacteria or the protozoa. This uncertainty, which is practically unimportant, may be ended any day, as active study of its nature is constantly going on under such masters as Metchnikoff, Roux, and others. Bloch, a high authority, calls it a protozoön.

Syphilis

Metchnikoff points out the fact that the female genital organs are the home of other forms of *Spirilla*, which may at times be mistaken for the *Spirochæte pallida*. Beside the *Spirochæte refringens* there is still another, the *Spirochæte balanitis*, and these, being sometimes found in lesions of syphilis, have been called secondary organisms.

The *Spirochæte pallida* is a delicate organism. It is smaller and slenderer than the other *Spirilla* mentioned, and has more spirils. It has been called "*pallida*," the pale *Spirochæte*, because of the technical difficulty of staining it for observation in laboratory work. Schaudinn, it is said, first named it *Spirochæte pallida*, later called it *Spirochæte pallidum*, and still later *Treponema pallidum*. The first name remains the one in general use.

It only survives for a few hours—six, Andrews says—outside of the human body. After that its infectious power is lost. It is destroyed by heating for an hour to 51 degrees Centigrade (124° Fahr. approximately). It needs moisture, and if dried dies quickly, but even with moisture present it is very perishable when removed from its human host. This readily perishable quality and early

8   Hygiene and Morality

loss of pathogenic power is of the highest importance in considering the subject of contagion by direct mechanical contact with infected objects, as will be seen later, and has a definite bearing on practical methods of disinfection and on the avoidance of direct infection from inanimate objects and personal contact.

So far, efforts to cultivate the *Spirochæte* in artificial media have not succeeded, but this, too, may be accomplished any day, as all the famous bacteriological laboratories of the world are experimenting on this line.

GENERAL RESULTS OF EXPERIMENTS. Experimental work so far has been successful in demonstrating the *Spirochæte pallida* in the primary, secondary, and tertiary lesions of syphilis; in the lymphatic organs and the lymph; in the saliva and urine; in arterial lesions; in the fœtus, and in the newborn congenitally syphilitic infant, which, indeed, always shows enormous numbers of the specific germ in its various organs.[1] It has also been occasionally demonstrated in the blood. Further, experimental work, chiefly that carried on in the Pasteur Institute under the

[1] Metchnikoff.

Syphilis

direction of Metchnikoff, and by Neisser in Java, has been successful in transmitting the disease syphilis to certain varieties of apes, and in thus clearing up some important and formerly unknown facts and principles that are of value for early and correct diagnosis and treatment.

Thus it has been shown that the virus of syphilis can be demonstrated in the internal organs within sixteen days after infection, and long before the usual time of appearance of the earliest outward sign of the disease, namely, the "primary sore."[1] Unremitting attempts made to obtain a prophylactic serum or mitigated virus such as has been successfully produced for diphtheria, tetanus, etc., have so far been only partially successful, but, though some scientists regard the production of such a serum or vaccine as a doubtful possibility, the efforts to produce it will no doubt go on until it has been accomplished.

The proof of the early extinction of the life of the germ after being removed from the body is one of the important results of experiment, and, in the work with apes, a number of data, valuable for diagnosis and treatment, have been secured, notably that of the "serum diagnosis" of Neisser,

[1] Neisser.

Wassermann, and Brink. This is based upon the natural reaction that takes place in the blood after the introduction of certain poisons, and the appearance in the blood of so-called "antibodies," or natural antagonists to the poison in question. These "antibodies," normally not demonstrable by ordinary methods of examination, may increase and be found in large quantities under the stimulus of the disease poison. Their presence in syphilis is now regarded as an important passive aid to diagnosis, though their absence would not necessarily prove the non-existence of the disease.

The effects of the drugs used in the clinical treatment of syphilis, especially mercury, have also been extensively and usefully studied in the course of animal experimentation.

SYMPTOMS AND COURSE OF SYPHILIS. Syphilis has been defined as a specific disease of slow evolution, propagated by inoculation (acquired syphilis), or by hereditary transmission (congenital syphilis).[1]

Acquired syphilis is invariably due to direct contact with the discharges or secretions of a patient already suffering from the disease. It is

[1] Osler.

Syphilis

supposed that some minute break or abrasion in the skin or mucous membrane exposed to the virus is a condition of infection, though this break may be too minute to be noticeable. The squamous epithelium seems to be the primary channel of infection. The germ of syphilis cannot be transmitted through the atmosphere in dust particles, as may happen in the case of the tubercle bacillus.

Syphilis is an infectious fever, running a slow or chronic course, and, like other fevers, it has a period of incubation followed by acute symptoms including skin eruptions and general disturbances of the health, and it has, later, sequelæ or remote consequences of definite and varied, often of frightful character. Unlike other fevers, which run their course in a few weeks, this one lasts for months and even for years, while its sequels, like those of scarlet fever, are permanent and terrible in their nature.

The course of syphilis is divided into three stages: primary, secondary, and tertiary.

PRIMARY STAGE. The primary stage begins with the close of the incubation period, while incubation itself may take from ten days to seven weeks after the time of exposure to infection. This variance in time is supposed to be due to the varying number of *Spirochæte pallida* present in the infectious material or discharges by which the disease is carried. The average period of incubation is three or four weeks. During this time there are no signs of disturbance, and the abrasion through which the poison has been received, heals.

Finally, at the end of the incubation period, a small red papule appears at the point of inoculation. It may or may not enlarge. A little later it breaks down in the centre, forming an ulcer, small or large as the case may be, but, as a rule, single. This is known as the "hard chancre," from the fact that the tissues about it are indurated and dense, with a gristle-like feeling, and it is known as the "primary lesion" or "initial sore" of syphilis. The discharge from this ulcer is highly contagious, yet, if the ulcer is of small size, it may be readily overlooked. In the primary stage there may be no disturbance of the general health, nor any symptoms that attract attention. The primary stage continues for from one to three months with no other signs of trouble than the primary lesion itself. This quiescent period is sometimes called the second incubation period.

Syphilis

At its close, rarely later than the twelfth week, an active set of constitutional symptoms come on.

SECONDARY STAGE. The poison has now been distributed by the lymphatic system, as evidenced by enlargement of the glands in all parts of the body. There may be fever, more or less marked and of variable character, and skin eruptions, also of very varied characteristics, the most usual being a rash resembling measles which appears first on the chest and abdomen, spreading thence to other parts of the body. One form of the eruption resembles smallpox; others bear resemblance to skin diseases of different origin and varying features. There is severe nocturnal headache and pain in the bones, with a general feeling of illness. The inner surfaces of the mouth and all the structures of the pharynx and throat may become sore, red, and swollen, sometimes so acutely so that solid food cannot be swallowed. The mucous patches which are among the most significant and special symptoms of syphilis may appear on all or any parts of the inner surfaces of the mouth and gums, tongue, tonsils, and pharynx. They may also appear at the corners of the lips, or in the nasal lining, or in the folds of the axillæ and the perineum, or even between the toes. The mucous patch is a flat, greyish ulcer, which secretes a copious, virulently infectious discharge. Other symptoms of the secondary stage are syphilitic iritis, inflammation of the periosteum and of the joints, alopecia, syphilitic onychia, and condylomata, or the "syphilitic warts" which are frequently found in the vulvar region. The labyrinth of the ear may be involved and deafness result.

TERTIARY STAGE. The oncoming of the tertiary stage cannot always be separated from the secondary stage by a definite line, nor can the symptoms of the secondary and tertiary periods always be distinctly separated in classification, as, in some cases, symptoms usually regarded as late ones may appear early, or, again, the stages may not run a perfectly typical course. Nor does the tertiary stage always develop. Tertiary symptoms, like sequels of other contagions, are not wholly inevitable. They may be averted by early, careful treatment carried on for a sufficient length of time.

When the third stage of syphilis does occur, its onset may not take place for months or even years after the primary sore. During a long

Syphilis

period the patient may have believed himself to be entirely well and free from danger. This slowness of development and insidious latency of the disease constitutes one of its most dread features. Andrews says: "No other communicable disease continues its manifestations after twenty and even fifty years after the original infection."

It is believed that the chief cause contributory to the development of tertiary symptoms is inadequate treatment in the very early stages. As a result of this inadequacy of care it may happen that cases which appeared mild and insignificant at the outset, and which, in consequence, may have received only brief or superficial treatment, develop most malignant and violent tertiary symptoms. There are, however, some cases where the virulence of the poison defies all, even early, treatment.

As a rule, the general condition of the patient and of his surroundings have much bearing upon the probable results of treatment. If the general health is good, surroundings sanitary, and treatment adequate and faithfully followed, the patient may generally feel hopeful of cure.

Alcoholism makes the prognosis much worse, and bad hygienic living conditions also add to a discouraging outlook. The parasites may not be actually killed, but only rendered latent and may, in consequence, produce tertiary symptoms at a remote period.

The typical characteristics of the third period of syphilis are "gummata" or soft tumors which may develop in any set of tissues, from the hard bony structure through the whole range of internal organs to the brain and skin. These tumors or gumma tend to ulceration and destruction of tissues, and produce the deformities sometimes seen, such as the destruction of the bridge of the nose, etc. Skin eruptions of a more formidable type than the earlier ones, and having a more pronounced tendency to ulcerate, appear in this stage.

CONGENITAL SYMPTOMS. Every feature of the acquired disease except the primary sore, says Dr. Osler, may be seen in the congenital form. The baby born with syphilis is wasted and withered, with the wrinkled "old" looking little face; fissures at the corners of the mouth; a discharge from the nostrils, "snuffles"; ulcerated lips; excoriated buttocks; dry and unhealthy skin; eruptions, especially about the extremities:

Syphilis

some or all of these symptoms may be present. The baby with these marked evidences of disease is not likely to live. Or, the baby may be born healthy looking and well, but after a few weeks' time may develop snuffles, eruptions, fissures about the mouth, loss of hair and eyebrows, or other less markedly characteristic symptoms. This process usually occurs between the third and twelfth week. Children with congenital syphilis, says Osler, rarely thrive. Certain ones may improve or recover, but there is apt to be a return of the disease at puberty. Even those who recover from the early symptoms do not develop normally. They often have a wizened, wasted look, their growth is slower, and there is a frequent condition known as "infantilism" which gives, for instance, to the youth of nineteen the appearance of a boy of twelve.

About the time of puberty, the child with inherited syphilis may develop persistent eye and ear diseases. Of all the organs of special sense, the eye is the one most frequently attacked. Disease of bones may appear early or late, and the late case of hereditary syphilis may display the dread gummata and end in general paresis. The lesions of the third stage are also infectious, though, as they are often situated in deep seated tissues, there is less opportunity for the infection to be conveyed to others.

The congenitally syphilitic infant is intensely infectious. Fournier says: "Nothing is so dangerous to its surroundings as a syphilitic infant."

SYPHILIS HEREDITARY IN THE LITERAL SENSE. Syphilis is hereditary, not in the sense of an inherited predisposition only, as is the case with tuberculosis (once believed to descend as an actual entity from one generation to another), but the disease itself may be inherited. In other words, the new-born baby may come into the world with the *Spirochæte pallida* present in enormous numbers in all or in any of its tissues. Morrow says: "Syphilis is the only disease which is transmitted in full virulence to the offspring."

HEREDITY TO THE THIRD GENERATION. It is a matter of some difference of opinion and controversy whether syphilis is transmissible to the third generation. The French school, fairly generally, some American writers, and Hutchinson, the English authority, take the negative, while many others withhold a positive pronounce-

Syphilis

ment. In the absence of a definite certainty, however, one cannot but recall the words of the Old Testament, "The sins of the fathers are visited upon the children, even unto the third and fourth generations," and surmise that they may reflect the accumulated wisdom of ages of experience. In this connection it may be remembered too that the exact study of syphilis is now, according to distinguished medical writers, only in its infancy.

It is supposed that, in a large number of cases, the syphilitic taint is derived from the father only; that the semen conveys the *Spirochæte pallida* directly to the product of conception. It is also authoritatively taught that, if the mother alone has transmitted the disease to the offspring the danger is graver—the fatality to the children more overwhelming than if the father alone has transmitted it. Recent studies emphasise the predominant part of the mother in heredity.

A phenomenon first pointed out by a noted surgeon of Dublin, Colles, and named after him, is that of a mother who, herself apparently free from the disease, gives birth to a child showing congenital taint, and can herself nurse her baby without becoming infected by it, whilst the most healthy wet-nurse nursing the same baby becomes infected. But it seems to be a question whether this mother, who appears to be immune, really is so or not. Osler speaks of her as receiving a "protective inoculation." Hutchinson makes the observation that it would be important to know how many such mothers showed tertiary symptoms in later life. This is at present not known, but he believes there is proof that there are many, and holds this to be corroborative of the view that such mothers really do receive an infection during pregnancy. The whole subject is one of present incertitude, and with further research is likely to be completely revised. Another phenomenon which has been called after Profeta is that of a child apparently healthy which nurses its syphilitic mother without becoming infected. This also must be taken with reserve as needing further exact investigation.

Finally, it is supposed that the offspring may escape infection altogether if the mother is not infected until late in pregnancy, especially if not until after the seventh month.

IMMUNITY. A study of the most recent writings gives the impression that it is regarded as, on the whole, doubtful whether a true natural immunity

Syphilis

against syphilis exists in the human individual. D'Arcy Power says that, as far as is now known, no healthy person is proof against syphilis, but that any one who is directly exposed to it, in the literal sense of having the *Spirochæte pallida* introduced into the lymphatic system, will contract the disease. Nor is there a certainty as to acquired immunity. Neisser holds that, in the case of syphilis, there is no such thing as the acquired immunity which is familiar as following upon some other contagious diseases—that is, when an individual, having once had a contagious disease and having been cured, is thereafter insusceptible to it. He teaches, as the result of his investigations with animals, that cases which appear to display immunity and resistance to fresh infection are really not cured, but have the *Spirochæte pallida* still present in their tissues, and that cases which had been really cured by treatment, *i. e.*, when the microscope proved that the *Spirochæte* had actually been killed, were susceptible to new infection.

While it is not always correct to make precise deductions from animal experimentation for man he believes that this is also true of human beings— that cases of so-called "immunity" are not such, but that these individuals still have the *Spirochæte pallida* present in their tissues. In October, 1908, he stated that no method of procuring active or passive immunity, nor mode of treatment with immunising substances, had been discovered.

On this point, Hutchinson says that he has seen seven cases of true second attacks of syphilis at intervals of from eighteen months to twelve years after the first attack. The possibility of a second attack, is therefore, he believes, only the expression of the efficiency of the treatment of the first. Lang of Vienna says that for a long time there was a belief in the absolute immunity conferred by a first attack of syphilis but that this belief was disproved by Zeissl and others. Reinfection, he holds, can only occur in individuals who have been perfectly cured. Those in whom the disease is still present are not susceptible to new infection.

Reinfected cases usually run a mild course. So, too, it is believed that races in which syphilis has long been widely prevalent show a less obvious type of symptom.

RELATION OF SYPHILIS TO THE NERVOUS SYS-

Syphilis

TEM. The relation of syphilis to a number of the disorders of the nervous system had only been imperfectly understood up to the time of the discovery of the *Spirochæte pallida*. Careful studies are now being pressed along this line, and it cannot be doubted that the rapid progress of modern medical science will continuously throw new light upon these obscure problems, to the incalculable benefit of the human race.

Some diseases of the nervous system are directly due to syphilis, as hemiplegia from syphilitic degeneration of the walls of arteries; and paralysis or convulsions due to syphilitic tumors of the brain or those lying at the roots of nerves.

Again, some of the most formidable nervous diseases, classed as para-syphilitic, are regarded not as in themselves syphilitic, but as resulting in some way from the virus of syphilis or from the changes it has brought about in the organs. Prominent among these are locomotor ataxia and the general paralysis of the insane. It was formerly held that the first mentioned disease might arise from other causes; that, though the great majority of cases were of definitely syphilitic origin, a certain percentage of the remainder must not be so regarded. But the more recent writers tend to the assumption that the syphilitic taint is invariably to be found in the previous history, even though it may be many years, or a full generation, earlier.[1]

THE RELATION OF SYPHILIS TO CARCINOMA. Recent writers point out the great importance of further investigation into the obscure relationship between syphilis and carcinoma. D'Arcy Power states that cancer is peculiarly liable to occur in the tissue which has undergone a chronic syphilitic inflammatory process, and speaks of the virus of syphilis as "preparing the tissues" for cancer, especially that form of it known as epithelioma. While there is no reason for supposing that syphilis is closely related to carcinoma yet its importance as a predisposing or favourable condition for the development of this terrible affliction should give added weight to every argument for the extirpation of syphilis from human society.

SYPHILIS AND TUBERCULOSIS. The author just quoted points out the inter-relation between syphilis and tuberculosis, and believes that

[1] Mott in *British Medical Journal*, Feb. 27, 1909.

Syphilis

syphilitic tissues are more liable to infection by the bacillus of tuberculosis than other equally ill-nourished tissues are, if syphilis-free. He emphasises the interaction between the two diseases, while, at a recent meeting of the American Society of Sanitary and Moral Prophylaxis the statement was made that, if syphilis could be wiped out, a vast amount of the tuberculosis now existent would also disappear.

SYPHILIS AND OTHER DISEASES. In a general way it may be stated that syphilis constitutes a predisposition to bear all other constitutional diseases badly. The intemperate, the tuberculous, the rheumatic, the malarial patient all suffer more, and find themselves in a less hopeful condition when syphilis or the syphilitic degeneration is present as a complication.

SYPHILIS AND ALCOHOLISM. A relationship or affinity appears to exist between syphilis, alcohol, and prostitution which unites them in a trio of great and evil menace to health. Dr. Morrow says:

Instruction would be incomplete without a warning as to the influence of alcohol in the instigation of immoral relations and as one of the most powerful auxiliaries of sexual contamination. The rôle of alcohol in the propagation of venereal diseases has not been sufficiently appreciated, and the consideration that every repressive measure against alcohol will be an important prophylactic measure against the spread of venereal diseases has not received the attention it deserves. Perhaps more than any other agency, alcohol relaxes the moral sense while it stimulates the sexual impulse.

Neisser speaks of "the fatal rôle of alcoholism which drives innumerable young men to exaggerated exercise of the sexual functions"; and Pontoppidan says:

> Alcohol is an inducing and even a downright cause of the rise and propagation of venereal diseases. Alcohol paralyses the will and understanding, and stimulates sexual and sentimental emotion. Abstinence and temperance movements must be taken as important allies in the prevention of venereal diseases.

Medical statistics show that an excessive proportion of venereal disease has been contracted while under the influence of alcohol. Dr. Forel's investigations suggest an affinity between syphilis and tissues that are habituated to alcohol. He finds that alcohol is oftener the exciting cause of infection in men than in women, while it oftener induces women to commit the first irregular act. Dr. Morrow states also that chronic alcoholism is a powerful factor in bringing on the development of severe and extensive lesions of the skin and mucous membranes; that it promotes the cerebral disorders of syphilis, and causes the disease to run into the third stage.

Loxton emphasises the necessity of cutting off alcohol entirely in the treatment of all venereal diseases, and cites cases of gonorrhœa where abrupt relapses with acute symptoms followed immediately after alcoholic drinks had been taken.[1]

Ravogli says:

Alcoholism when associated with syphilis is also a most important factor in crime. We know the deleterious influence of alcohol in individuals affected with syphilis,—so much so that the French speak of a special kind of syphilis, *la syphilis alcoholisée*. Some writers indeed go so far as to claim that the general paralyses of tertiary syphilis only occur in those who have been addicted to drink.

SYPHILIS AND CRIME. A suggestive article by Ravogli on syphilis in relation to crime gives the scientific reasons of the author for believing

[1] *British Medical Journal*, Feb. 27, 1909.

that the injurious action of the syphilitic virus upon the vascular system and the structures of nerves is an explanation of much of the degeneracy that is evidenced by crime, and especially by cruel and persecutory kinds of crime where the perpetrator enjoys the sufferings of others. He quotes Barthélemy, who says that "the great class of heredo-syphilitics forms the ranks of the degenerate, unbalanced, obnubilated mattoids," and that this heredity, with alcoholism, is the most effective cause of human degradation. Ravogli says: "The existence of moral insanity admits of no doubt, and that it is often the result of syphilitic alterations of blood-vessels is easy to demonstrate."

While he does not mean to be understood as saying that syphilis is the determining cause of crime, he does believe that it is one of the predisposing factors of crime, and he then goes on to say:

A strange relation exists between syphilis, crime, and prostitution—cases of prostitution which cannot be explained by poverty or by special accident have to be attributed to hereditary syphilis. Prostitution and crime go hand in hand, and in the families where the brothers are criminals the sisters are pros-

Syphilis

titutes. Syphilis is the tie between crime and prostitution when it causes the affections of the nervous system resulting in moral degeneration.

STATISTICAL ESTIMATES OF SYPHILIS. No comprehensive or general system of counting the cases of syphilis or the other venereal disorders is yet officially established in any country. The available statistics, therefore, being those collected by medical specialists in their own practice and in hospital records, though authoritative, and sufficiently startling, have not the extent of those collected by public bureaus or health departments. Nevertheless there are data enough to enable medical experts to make very definite assertions as to the prevalence of venereal diseases and their share in morbidity and mortality.

The general prevalence of syphilis is estimated at from five to eighteen per cent. of populations, some countries having a worse record than others. It is stated in medical writings that from ten to fifteen per cent. of the male population of Europe have syphilis.

Destruction of the fœtus and a heavy infant mortality are prominent results of syphilis. Morrow says: "No disease has such a murderous

Hygiene and Morality

influence upon the offspring." It is known that syphilis is responsible for a large percentage of all miscarriages, while the death-rate of congenitally syphilitic infants is described by the expression "Poly-Mortality."

Figures taken from European hospital records and from physicians' note-books, all classes of the community being considered as one, show a double fatality when both parents are infected, or an infant death-rate of sixty-eight per cent. In private practice only, the social status here being rather superior, the infant mortality is sixty or sixty-one per cent. Free public hospitals, where the most indigent cases find refuge, show the worst figures, from eighty-four to eighty-six deaths in every hundred infants. One in every four or five lives long enough to pass the heritage on. Physicians record instances of the extinction of entire families from syphilis. Fournier cites one such case, where, to 157 births, there were 157 deaths from this cause. In the *Transactions* of the American Society of Sanitary and Moral Prophylaxis the statement is made that in France alone syphilis kills twenty thousand children annually. The ages at which syphilis is, in a large proportion of cases, contracted, give melancholy testimony

Syphilis

to the prevalent neglect of the young. There are authentic medical figures showing that from thirty to forty per cent. of the cases of this disease are infected between the ages of fourteen and twenty years.

Besides the hereditary infection of children by their parents the infection of wives by their husbands is common. Morrow's records show that, of all the women suffering from syphilis who attended the clinics of a large hospital, seventy per cent. were respectable married women who had been infected by their husbands. He says further that "possibly ten per cent. of men who marry infect their wives with venereal disease," and his estimation of the total number of syphilitics in the United States is two million.

It is believed that, generally speaking, about ten per cent. of all cases of syphilis are transmitted accidentally in various ways like ordinary contagions, that is to say, not by sexual contact. Thus, of 887 cases of syphilis in women, recorded by Fournier, 842 had been acquired in sexual contact, while the others had been accidentally conveyed by ordinary contact, through instruments, tubes, utensils, etc., or by caring for or suckling diseased infants, etc.

THE SOURCE AND SPREAD OF SYPHILIS. A distinction must be made between (a) cause; (b) source or breeding-place; (c) mode of spread of any infectious disease.

The cause of every such disease is a special micro-organism. The sources or breeding-places where these organisms flourish and congregate vary, as we know, while the means by which they are disseminated broadcast also vary, almost to infinity.

Those contagions that are called, familiarly, filth diseases, do not cease being filth diseases when they are conveyed into clean homes to strike down cleanly living individuals. In the study of every infectious disease knowledge of the breeding-place or native haunt of its germ is of the utmost importance for practical hygiene. Thus the world has rung with the announcements of the mosquito carriers of yellow fever and malaria and with the exploits of those medical heroes who sacrificed their lives in the search for this knowledge;—again, in the case of tuberculosis, information as to the breeding-places and modes of dissemination of the tubercle bacillus is published in public places, told in public lectures, and, indeed, almost cried in the streets.

Syphilis

In the case of typhoid fever, it is accepted by all intelligent people as a civic crime to neglect water supplies. So in the case of every infectious germ; as its habitat and ways of spreading are learned, the knowledge is given freely and fully to the world. In the case of syphilis, and of other venereal diseases as well, though their specific micro-organisms have not long been identified, their breeding-places and most prominent mode of transmission have been well known for many years by the medical and legal professions and by sophisticated members of the laity, but, because of the perplexing, complicated, and difficult social web in which they were woven, these facts have been concealed and an absolutely opposite policy has prevailed from that followed, for instance, with tuberculosis. With the latter, full publicity: with the former, until most recently, almost unbroken secrecy. Every one talks of tuberculosis; almost no one of venereal disease. It is true that tuberculosis also was not made a matter of public, national importance until its curable, preventable, and non-inheritable nature was discovered. This gives hope for believing that venereal diseases also may be brought into the open, since it can be shown that they are not only curable, but, more than any others, preventable, since their prevention may be a matter of choice and of the individual will. To these hopeful facts the certainty of the relentless hereditary transmission of syphilis should act as a powerful spur.

BREEDING-PLACE OF SYPHILIS AND THE VENEREAL DISEASES. The breeding-place of all venereal diseases without exception is in the social institution called prostitution, or sexual promiscuity: in the debasement and degradation of what should be the highest and most revered of physical powers, those involved in the act of generation. Bred and cultivated in prostitution, venereal diseases spread thence through the community, attacking the innocent as well as the guilty, the pure as well as the impure, just as typhoid fever is no respecter of persons, no matter how strict their own personal sanitary standards may be.

How, or why, the parasitic powers of the *Spirochæte pallida* first declared themselves in unlawful, not in lawful sexual intercourse, is a mystery. But it is certain that this organism is never met with in the relation of marriage unless it has been brought from with-

Syphilis

out. Excesses in the marriage relation, though productive of other evils, do not bring on venereal diseases. If, as some writers state, even polygamy does not promote them, then it would seem as if the original exciting cause favourable to the parasitic vigour of the *Spirochæte pallida* must have been in some way related to the numbers and variety of male beings who practised a heterogeneous promiscuity. Howsoever their derivation might be traced, prostitution is now as certainly the abiding-place and inexhaustible source of this as of other germs of venereal disease, as the marshy swamp is the abode of the malaria-carrying mosquito, or the polluted water supply of the typhoid bacillus. Pontoppidan of Copenhagen says: "Even if contagion is carried in different ways, its origin can nearly always be traced back to prostitution." And Bulkley says: "Prostitution undoubtedly stands foremost as a cause of syphilis and far outweighs all other causes together." Again, he says: "In the enormous majority of cases syphilis is acquired in illicit intercourse." Osler says, "Inextricably blended with it [the social evil] is the prevention of syphilis." Morrow speaks of "The original source of these infections

36   Hygiene and Morality

in that irregular commerce between the sexes known as prostitution."

Since the discovery of the germ of syphilis there appears some tendency on the part of some medical writers to remove syphilis from the list of venereal diseases. As has been mentioned, it is frequently classified separately, thus: "Syphilis and the Venereal Diseases." The argument is that, with the fuller knowledge of its many modes of transmission, its constitutional features, and hereditability, its venereal stigma should be removed. Yet, as, although a germ disease, its germ does not appear to be distributed generally, like the pus-producing germs; as the disease syphilis never breaks out afresh under normal conditions, nor develops from the germ in the course of moral living, but is cultivated in morally unclean sexual relations, then it does not seem incorrect to call it a venereal disease, even though it may be communicated to moral and innocent individuals in non-venereal ways arising in the ordinary contact of daily life. The important things to know are: That it is cultivated in prostitution and thence spread through the community in ways which are to be mentioned in detail. These ways are classified by Bulkley as follows:

Syphilis

I. Inherited. II. Marital. III. Extra-genital.

I. The hereditary communicability of syphilis has been discussed.

II. The marital mode of transmission is the infection of one partner (usually the wife) by the other during the performance of the act of generation. As this act offers the most favourable possible opportunity for infection of such a nature to be carried, it results that by far the greatest proportion of cases that are innocently or accidentally received—a proportion that is variably estimated—have been conveyed in the marriage relation.

III. With the knowledge of the micro-organism and its presence in all syphilitic lesions and in the discharges from primary sores, ulcers, mucous patches, secretions of the mouth and nose, etc., it may be readily understood that the opportunities for infection to be conveyed in the ordinary processes of daily life, especially when people live under crowded or uncleanly conditions, are very numerous.

That syphilis is not more frequently conveyed by incidental contact than is actually the case is due to the, fortunately, very short life of the germ outside the human body.

All of the common acts of daily life may serve as means of infection during the brief period of the parasite's existence, viz., eating and drinking from cups and saucers, knives, forks, and spoons that may have been in contact with the lips of a syphilitic; putting pencils, pins, money, whistles, or any other article in the mouth after it may possibly have been in that of an infected person.

Towels, handkerchiefs, pillow-cases, or any article of bedding as well as water-closet seats and bath-tubs may serve as carriers. Surgical and dental instruments, shaving apparatus, medical appliances in familiar use, as bulbs, sprays, douche bags, spatulas, and syringes, may convey the poison. Cases have been recorded where it has been inoculated during the process of vaccination, and occasional known instances of this kind have had much to do with strengthening the objections of anti-vaccinationists and intensifying the popular prejudice against vaccination that is found in some communities. Syphilis has also been conveyed in circumcision and other slight operations.

Laundresses and rag-pickers have not infrequently been infected by soiled or cast-off clothing;

Syphilis

physicians and surgeons are always liable to this danger in the course of their professional work; midwives are exposed during the delivery and care of patients; nurses have been infected while caring for patients, the nature of whose illness had not been made known to them, and with whom they were therefore not as vigilantly on guard as they should have been.

Most dangerous of all the avenues of accidental infection is contact with the person of the syphilitic, on account of the probability of then receiving germs that are living and virulent. Any such contact with the lips, teeth, or tongue is especially dangerous, such as kissing (an act which is known to have been the cause of many innocent cases), playful biting or mouthing (such as is often carried on playfully between children and adults), sucking wounds, licking with the tongue, etc.

The syphilitic baby is an especially infectious object because of the many necessities of the baby for close personal care and handling in feeding and bathing it.

CHAPTER II

GONORRHŒA AND CHANCROID

GONORRHŒA; ITS SPECIFIC MICRO-ORGANISM. Gonorrhœa is caused by an organism called *Gonococcus gonorrhœæ* which was discovered by Neisser in 1879 and has been especially studied and described by Bumm. As it is usually seen in pairs, it is also called the *Diplococcus gonorrhœæ* or the *Micrococcus* of Neisser. It is cultivable with difficulty, and does not survive many transplantations, yet transplanting does not lessen its virulence. It is always found in gonorrhœal pus, but is never found in other inflammatory conditions unless these are of gonorrhœal origin. It is said to perish quickly in sunlight and to be killed in a few hours by drying. Experimentation with it in the inoculation of animals has been attended with special and unusual difficulties.

The *Gonococcus gonorrhœæ* can live for years, or indefinitely, in the human tissues in a dormant

Gonorrhœa and Chancroid 41

or latent state, latent gonorrhœa being frequent in both men and women. This characteristic, unknown until the day of bacteriological study with the microscope, and not immediately discovered even then, gives the disease a specially uncertain character and makes it quite as treacherous as syphilis, if not even more so.

After remaining latent for a long time, perhaps for years, the organism of gonorrhœa, if conveyed to the sound and healthy tissues of another individual (such tissues being spoken of, in regard to the organism, as "virgin," or "sterile" tissues), finds its most favourable conditions for growth and then excites an actively acute inflammation and displays its utmost virulence.

HISTORY OF GONORRHŒA. Gonorrhœa is primarily a genito-urinary disease, and was formerly believed to be a purely local affection. It is supposed to be as old as the human race, and, like syphilis, its main line of propagation has always been in the promiscuous intercourse of prostitution, whence it has been disseminated in every direction. Ancient writings specify its symptoms with enough exactitude to make its identity plain. This identity was lost in the epidemic of syphilis in the 15th century, to which allusion has been made. During the 18th century the difference between syphilis and gonorrhœa might have been rediscovered, had not an inexact experiment of the celebrated John Hunter caused the medical profession to regard all venereal diseases as one up to the time of the work of Ricord.

If syphilis has only been fairly well understood for the last half-century, gonorrhœa, at least in so far as women are concerned, has only been estimated according to its real gravity in the last decade, though Neisser made his discovery in 1879. In 1857 two medical writers, Bernitz and Goupil, had made studies of gonorrhœal infection of the Fallopian tubes, but had found no followers. In 1878 Noeggerath sounded a warning, declaring that individuals with gonorrhœa could remain infectious during a lifetime, but he was regarded as an alarmist and his statistics of the frequency of gonorrhœa in married men as exaggerations. Gonorrhœa had been regarded as an ordinary "catarrhal" inflammation of the mucous membrane, locating itself usually in the urethra, and as, in men, the disease was well known to be acquired in promiscuous sex relations, it was commonly regarded with indifference, or

Gonorrhœa and Chancroid

even with levity, as a proof of rakishness, the purulent discharge being colloquially described in military countries as the "goutte militaire."

In the light of modern knowledge of the disastrous part taken by the *gonococcus* of gonorrhœa in that sad array of obscure and unnecessary ailments which have been erroneously called "Diseases of Women," the traces of this levity make painful reading, found, as they are, even in medical writings of a generation ago or less. To-day, instead of being regarded as a local disease, gonorrhœa also, like syphilis, is known to develop constitutional disturbances of a serious and chronic nature, and suggestions are not wanting that the former point of view will soon be antiquated.

COURSE AND SYMPTOMS OF GONORRHŒA. Osler divides the course of gonorrhœa into three stages:

1. Primary infection.
2. Extension through the entire genito-urinary tract.
3. Systemic infection.

PRIMARY INFECTION. The period of infection is from twelve hours to a week or more, the average being one or two days. In adults the urethra is usually the point of infection, or, in women, it may be also the cervix uteri, for the reason that the delicate linings of these parts are only weakly resistant and are easily penetrated by the bacillus. The uninjured squamous epithelium of the adult is not easily infected. With little girls, infection usually attacks the vulva and vagina, by reason of their delicate structure in childhood.

The symptoms of the primary stage are those of an ordinary acute local infection, with itching and burning of the parts, redness and swelling, pains, often intense, on urination, and a discharge, first mucous and finally purulent, with œdema of the surrounding tissues, excoriations, multiple abscesses, and perhaps hemorrhage from swollen papillæ. To the eye there is nothing to distinguish the symptoms from those of an ordinary inflammation, and only the microscope makes the diagnosis positive. Formerly, it was believed that cure had taken place when the discharge ceased. It is now known that this is far from being the case.

SECOND STAGE. The inflammation now goes on and involves the organs of generation and the urinary tract, ascending the ureters and

Gonorrhœa and Chancroid

spreading, it may be, to the kidneys, where it may produce a fatal pyelitis. In women a large proportion of all cases of cystitis, salpingitis, metritis, ovaritis, and pelvic peritonitis, as well as many cases of infection after childbirth are caused by the *gonococcus*.

The most serious, because irreparable, action of gonorrhœa upon the organs of generation is to cause sterility in both men and women. The frequency with which this sequel occurs will be referred to under "Statistics." In women this sterility is sometimes brought about by occlusion or blocking of the Fallopian tubes. Again, there is what is called "one-child sterility." When this happens, the *gonococcus*, at first restricted in its location to the cervix uteri, is enabled owing to the relaxation of the parts after childbirth, to extend to the tubes and ovaries. Or, again, the necessity of complete operative removal of all the female organs of generation effectually puts an end to all expectations of maternity.

THE DESTRUCTION OF EYESIGHT. Calamitous as are the sequels of gonorrhœa to the adult, especially to the married woman, no other single effect wrought by it can compare with the tragedy of infants, blinded at birth by virulent gonorrhœal poison, which enters the eyes during the infant's passage through the vaginal canal. This, too, will be referred to under "Statistics." Gonorrhœal poison is most actively destructive of the cornea, and the danger of incurring blindness from having the eyes infected with pus or discharge containing this virus is equally as great for adults as for infants. The opportunity for infection is less, yet blindness of older children and adults from the *gonococcus* received from towels, sheets and pillow-cases, fingers, handkerchiefs, etc., is frequent, and cases have occurred where nurses have lost one or both eyes through lack of sufficient precautions.

THIRD STAGE. The constitutional forms of gonorrhœa include, besides disease of the kidneys already mentioned, gonorrhœal arthritis, an intractable and obstinate form of rheumatism, prone to relapses, and gonorrhœal endocarditis. These are regarded as its two most serious constitutional sequels. There is also a gonorrhœal septicæmia. Authorities mention a urogenital tuberculosis, to which chronic urethritis has the relation of a predisposing cause. Morrow speaks of

Gonorrhœa and Chancroid   47

this as a recent acquisition of knowledge, and adds that modern investigations are showing that it is possible for the *gonococcus* to be taken up by the blood and lymph and carried to all organs of the body, and that it may affect them all injuriously. It has been found in the brain and cord, the pleura, the liver, spleen, and kidneys, the endocardium, the sheaths of tendons and of joints, and in the periosteum. Finally, it may not be amiss to place under the constitutional effects of the *gonococcus* that innumerable army of chronically semi-invalided married women of all ages, who, without having clearly defined loss of health, "have never been well since married," whose whole existence is a drag and who have often failed to find the commiseration due them, this having indeed been oftener given to the husbands, whose lot in having ailing wives was all unknowingly due, in many cases, to their own transmission to these unsuspecting and unfortunate women of the deadly *gonococcus* of Neisser.

MODES OF TRANSMISSION. Though in the majority of cases the germ is conveyed during the act of coitus, it is also possible for it to be carried in the contact of daily life, and it is only the brevity of its existence after being dried that saves many cases from infection. Infection from unclean water-closet seats is frequent, instances having been known where a whole series of cases of vulvo-vaginitis have arisen from this cause. It is pointed out by medical writers that it is not necessary to conclude that little girls with a gonorrhœal discharge have been violated or addicted to bad practices (though such may have been the case) as it is quite possible for them to have contracted the disease from badly kept school closets, or from sleeping in the same bed and being contaminated by the sheets or clothing of diseased persons. Family towels under such circumstances are sources of danger, and public baths and tubs are also known to have been media of contagion.

IMMUNITY AND ANTI-SERUM TREATMENT. It is not believed that there is immunity against the *gonococcus*. Serum treatment has been tried in certain forms of constitutional disease, and beneficial results have been claimed in the case of rheumatism. The Lister Institute prepares an "Anti-gonococcus Vaccine," which is a preparation of dead *gonococci* that is said to be poisonous

Gonorrhœa and Chancroid

to the living germ.[1] It is probably too early to find anything quite authoritative upon this line of study.

The statistics of gonorrhœa are so startling as to seem almost incredible. Like those of syphilis, they are drawn from the records of hospitals and medical practitioners, as health boards ignore the existence of venereal diseases.

PREVALENCE OF GONORRHŒA. Morrow quotes Neisser to the effect that gonorrhœa is the most widespread and universal of diseases in the adult male. European records indicate that about seventy-five per cent. of all men have gonorrhœa.

Assuming that a somewhat better moral standard prevails in the United States, it is given as a conservative estimate that the prevalence of both gonorrhœa and syphilis among men is at least sixty per cent. Morrow says that it is impossible to estimate accurately the extent to which gonorrhœa is conveyed to wives in marriage, but that it is generally agreed that this is greater than is generally suspected. Statistics gathered in New York City by the Committee of Seven indicated

[1] *British Medical Journal*, Feb. 27, 1909.

that nearly thirty per cent. of all venereal diseases of women in that city had been transmitted in marriage by the husbands. The remainder (leaving out hereditary transmission and accidental infection) would probably be found among prostitutes. As to these unfortunate centres of infection, J. Taber Johnson estimates, conservatively, that at least thirty per cent. of their whole mortality is due to gonorrhœa.

STERILITY. Neisser regards gonorrhœa as responsible for more than forty-five per cent. of sterile marriages, while Morrow points out that these figures refer to primary, not to secondary sterility, which is additional. Gonorrhœa is the foremost cause of male sterility. One specialist found thirty cases of male sterility in ninety-six sterile marriages, while the statement is made by Morrow that men are ultimately responsible for from fifty to seventy-five per cent. of all sterility in married life. In from twenty to twenty-five per cent. of such cases, the husband is sterile. In the others, he has infected the wife, making her sterile.

The extent of secondary sterility is not known. A major share, then, of all sterility is to be laid at the door of the *gonococcus*.

Gonorrhœa and Chancroid 51

DISEASES OF WOMEN. The responsibility of the *gonococcus* in causing these diseases is variably estimated by different surgeons, ranging from forty to eighty per cent. All cases of pus in the Fallopian tubes are gonorrhœal, while at least fifty per cent. of all gynæcological operations are necessita ed by the *gonococcus*. This is a conservative estimate, some gynæcologists giving figures from their own practice that are much higher.

BLINDNESS. Eighty per cent. of all the purulent ophthalmia of infants is gonorrhœal, and from fifteen to twenty-five per cent. of all the blindness in America is due to the same cause. Neisser says that Germany alone has 30,000 blind persons whose affliction was caused by gonorrhœal pus, while in Paris the institutions for the blind show that forty-five per cent. of the cases have been due to this infection.

SUMMARY OF SYPHILIS AND GONORRHŒA. The consensus of expert medical opinion is, that, as a depopulating factor, gonorrhœa is more formidable than syphilis, and that it is also more perilous to the wife. Syphilis is more destructive to the life of offspring; gonorrhœa more destructive to the female organs of generation and to the general health. The hereditary quality and slow development of syphilis constitute its chief terrors, but the treacherous nature and persistent vitality of the *gonococcus* make gonorrhœa almost, if not quite, as terrible. Syphilis is, as a rule, more curable. The prognosis of gonorrhœa is always most uncertain. Both show certain types which are believed to be incurable.

Taking them together, they seem to exhibit the true race suicide, and both, says Taber Johnson, are intimately connected with the degeneration of races and the downfall of nations. Grandin says: "Man, largely through ignorance of the calamities following the misuse of this [the reproductive] instinct, has converted it into one for the extermination of the species."

CHANCROID (VENEREAL SORE; SOFT CHANCRE). The identity of the specific micro-organism of this last of the venereal diseases is still uncertain. A strepto-bacillus called the bacillus of Ducrey has been demonstrated in the soft chancre but it has not been proved to be its sole or specific cause.

Gonorrhœa and Chancroid

Clinically, Bassereau, in 1856, determined that chancroid and syphilis were not the same. Nevertheless mistakes in confusing the two were frequently made until the organism of syphilis was discovered.

Venereal sore is by far the simplest and least dangerous of the three diseases under consideration. If treated promptly it is readily curable, though, if neglected, serious complications may ensue and cure be a more difficult matter. The incubation period is short; from several hours to several days. The first manifestation is a small nodule which proceeds rapidly toward suppuration, forming a painful ulcer with an intensely infectious discharge. The ulcer is deep and irregular, and its tendency is to spread and become multiple. Herein lies the danger of complications. Neglected ulcers may involve the glands and other parts in their vicinity with much consequent destruction of tissues locally, but the disease has no constitutional complications, nor has it sequels or belated manifestations. If properly treated from the outset, from four to six weeks suffice for cure. It only runs a prolonged course when neglected.

Venereal sore is always located on the genitalia.

SOURCES OF MATERIAL USED IN THE PREPARATION OF PART I

Bloch, Ivan, Der Ursprung der Syphilis. Jena, 1901.
Bolduan, Charles Frederick, M.D., Immune Sera (Appendix A: Serum Diagnosis of Syphilis). New York, 1908.
Bulkley, L. D., M.D., Syphilis in the Innocent. New York, 1894.
Bull, Ophthalmia Neonatorum and its Prophylaxis. In New York Medical Journal, May 15, 1909.
Findlay, Palmer, M.D., Gonorrhœa in Women. 1908.
Forel, August, M.D., Alcohol and Questions of Sex. In Report of the International Congress against Alcohol. 1905.
Forel, August, M.D., Alkohol und venerische Krankheiten. In Report of the International Congress against Alcohol, 1901.
Fournier, Alfred, Syphilis et Mariage. Paris, 1890.
Fournier, Alfred, Traité de la Syphilis. 1903.
Francke, Hermann, M.D., Beitrag zur Entwickelung bösartiger Geschwülste auf dem Boden alter Syphilitischer Narben. Würzburg, 1894.
Horaud, Réné Denis, M.D., Syphilis et Cancer. Lyon, 1907.
Johnson, J. Taber, M.D., The Influence of Gonorrhœa as a Factor in Depopulation. In Journal of the American Medical Association, August 10, 1907.
Metchnikoff, Élie, The Microbiology of Syphilis. In A System of Syphilis. Edited by D'Arcy Power and J. Keogh Murphy. London, 1908.
Morrow, Prince A., M.D., Gonorrhœæ Insontium, especially in Relation to Marriage. In New York Medical Journal, June 27 and July 4, 1903.
Morrow, Prince A., M.D., Prognosis and Relation of Syphilis

Sources of Material Used 55

to Marriage and Heredity. In Medical News, Sept. 2, 1907.

Morrow, Prince A., M.D., Social Diseases and Marriage. New York, 1905.

Mott, Syphilis. In British Medical Journal, Feb. 27, 1909.

Noeggerath, Emil, M.D., Die latente Gonorrhöe im weiblichen Geschlecht. Tr. Amer. Gyn. Soc. I. 1876.

Osler, William, M.D., Practice of Medicine. [Syphilis and Gonorrhœa.] London and New York, 1909.

Pontoppidan, Erik, M.D., What Venereal Diseases Mean and How to Prevent Them. Translated by W. Jessen.

Ravogli, Syphilis in Relation to Crime. In Ohio State Medical Journal, August, 1906.

Rogers and Torrey, The Treatment of Gonorrhœal Infection by a Specific Antitoxin. In Journal of the American Medical Association, Sept. 14, 1907.

System of Medicine, A. [Syphilis, etc.] Edited by Allbutt. London, 1906.

System of Syphilis, A. [Several Authors.] Edited by D'Arcy Power and J. Keogh Murphy. London, 1906.

Taylor, Prognosis in Syphilis. In Medical News, Sept. 2, 1907.

Torrey, An Antigonococcus Serum. In Journal of the American Medical Association, Jan. 27, 1906.

Part II. Prostitution

CHAPTER I

CONTROL AND REGULATION OF PROSTITUTION

THERE is a long and revolting history of the spasmodic attempts made from time to time during the past ages to control or punish prostitution. These attempts usually took the form of grotesque and brutal punishments for women, rarely for men. As a rule, the vicious male seems to have been overlooked or regarded as an insignificant factor in the problem. Punishments meted out to the woman were chiefly hypocritical or vindictive, not in the least preventive. Sometimes she was put into an iron cage and dipped into the river,—almost but not quite drowned; sometimes her nose was cut off; or she was whipped or compelled to wear a distinguishing dress. She has always been the victim of blackmail, and the methods by which this has been levied show a remarkable similarity right down through the ages to modern times: they were usually the enactment of non-preventive legislation, of a petty and harassing character, with the imposition of heavy fines for breach of observance. As such legislation simply made it more difficult for her to earn her bread in the only way open to her, it of course had to be violated, and the fines collected were divided between the accuser and the city government. Perhaps this mode of profit-sharing is not yet obsolete. It is needless to give much time to the painful details of centuries that are gone, and it will suffice to state simply that all such legislation rested, as it still does, on the acceptance (once unquestioned, but to-day no longer so) of the double standard of morals.

THE DOUBLE MORAL STANDARD. The essential feature of the double code or standard of morals is the entire absence of logical sequence. Therefrom results the injustice which is so striking, both from the standpoint of reason and of humanity.

The double standard tacitly permits men to indulge freely and unchecked in sexual irregularity without consequent loss of social standing, but it dooms the women who are necessarily involved in these irregularities to social ostracism and even to complete degradation.

In order to justify immoral practices among themselves and to have a plausible explanation ready if criticism offered, the doctrine of "physical necessity" has been invented for men by themselves, and has even been fortified by the positive teachings of prominent medical men. This doctrine, however, has never been extended to women, but, instead, the cowardly and cruel theory of innate depravity has been industriously disseminated as applying to "fallen women," thus skilfully ensuring an isolated position for these unfortunates, and effectually checking the outgrowth of pity for them among women of the protected classes. The practical results of this psychological jugglery have been, that, of two partners in one and the same act, neither one of whom could execute this act alone, and with whom, if the element of compulsion entered as a complication, it could not possibly be present in the case of the stronger partner,—men, the stronger, have remained free from blame; women, the weaker, have lived under a curse.

The fact that this way of regarding the woman concerned disproves the argument of "physical necessity" is only a part of the illogicality of the whole. It is evident that, if unregulated sexual practice were really necessary for men, there could be no element of shame or wrong in it, and there could therefore, obviously, be none for the women, for no act that is physically necessary is wrong, no matter how primal it may be.

In order to give strength to the social structure of prostitution, certain catch phrases have been passed current to act as mental hypnotics. For instance: "Prostitution must always exist, because it always has existed. Because it always has existed, therefore it always must exist." But it will be seen that, in company with this dictum, there have always gone very definite social and legal contrivances for ensuring its existence.

MODERN SYSTEMS OF REGULATION. In spite of the hitherto generally accepted belief in the necessity and right of men to practise sexual irregularity, the presence of prostitution in the community, though the inevitable result of such practice, has been regarded as a "social evil," partly because of its accompaniment of disease. In order to minimise the danger of disease while maintaining prostitution, associations of men have, in the past, set

Control of Prostitution 63

themselves to the task of making vice safe, by establishing systems of "Regulation" with medical inspection of female prostitutes. This device originated, it is said, with Napoleon Bonaparte, who thought it proper that women should be sacrificed to his soldiers, but did not wish the soldiers to be invalided. Since his day, regulatory systems have been established in most European countries. They vary somewhat in detail, and have been roughly divided into three types: the Scandinavian, the simplest and the most free from obnoxious features, combining a certain amount of police supervision with the compulsory reporting of venereal diseases and ample free medical service without a stigma attached to it; the German, sometimes called Neisser's system, highly complicated, with some slight attempt at more logic than is found in the third, called the unilateral system, and which has been adopted in many foreign countries, having reached its most notorious development in France, where, in the main, it is still in force, though it is probable that its downfall is near.

Opposed alike to all systems of state or police regulation of prostitution are the principles of the abolitionists, to be discussed later, and of the most modern and wisest socio-medical teachers.

The organisation of the unilateral system was as follows: A special department of police, called Morals Police (*Police des Mœurs*), was authorised to regulate and control prostitution as, in general, the head of the department saw fit; that is, ordinarily no public legislation defined their powers, but these were defined in police codes and in municipal ordinances. At the very outset, therefore, the women thus dealt with were excluded from the realm of the common law. The police had full power to arrest any women whom they might "believe" or "suspect," or "have reason to think" were immoral. This part of their powers rested chiefly upon a spy system of plain-clothes men, and anonymous letters were regarded as valuable sources of information. Arrest was followed by forcible medical examination, and the woman's name and address were inscribed on the lists in the police department. Every two weeks, or at other specified times, she was compelled to appear for examination, and, if found diseased, was confined in what was essentially a hospital prison.

The one-time head of the Morals Police of

Control of Prostitution

Paris, when asked wherein lay the chief strength of his system, replied: "Arrests; always arrests; more and more arrests; that is our only hope:"

That innocent women were often subjected to arrest and even imprisonment under this system was regarded as an unavoidable incident.

The unfortunates under police surveillance could never hope to escape from their life. Hounded by the police wherever they went, their outlook was described by Dr. Mireur, a defender of the system, in these words:

Cut off, not only from society but from heaven; from hope, and from the power to repent; nevertheless [he added] inscription and licensing are essential, indispensable, even as prostitution itself.

All systems of regulation alike brought into existence the licensed or "tolerated" houses of ill-fame, and such houses were protected by the police. Their keepers possessed a certain status by reason of this connection, and the appearance of recognition and support by the government confused the moral sense of the people. The keepers of such places have always been active supporters of regulative acts, because the women are then more completely helpless. A German chief of police admitted in his reports that the inscription of prostitutes by the police aggravated their abject condition in a horrible manner, while a member of the Reichstag once said: "It is well known that these are marked women and can never reform."

Such is the system, which, with varying modifications and with some differences of detail as to the harshness with which it has been or is enforced, still prevails widely under the general term, "The Continental System of the Regulation of Vice." It has recently been discarded in Italy, and has been strongly condemned by public commissions in France. Switzerland has given it up, except in Geneva, where it is in force in full ignominy.

It seems almost incredible that there are many who would willingly see this system implanted in the United States. More than one attempt has been made to introduce it into this country, and arguments in its favour are not infrequently heard. It is for this reason, among others, that women should be informed and alert upon a subject which would otherwise seem too horrible to contemplate.

The continental system of licensed houses of

Control of Prostitution

ill-fame, as will be seen in a later chapter, has been the breeder for the white slave traffic, and these houses have been the main market of the traders and have afforded the trade its security. The unfortunate women hate the licensed houses because of their tyrannous features, and it has never been easy to fill the vacancies caused by disease and death. An organised system of supply and demand has therefore grown up, having developed early in the 19th century, not very long after the establishment of the regulation system. It must be explained that no government has ever consciously encouraged a white slave trade, but this has been the logical though unforeseen result of giving the tolerated houses a recognised status.

THE INTRODUCTION OF STATE REGULATION INTO GREAT BRITAIN. The strongest bulwark of regulated vice in all countries has been the military element. It has been a generally accepted understanding that armies of men must have free access to abandoned women, and it has always been a subject of serious concern with authorities to make this vice as safe as possible, in order that the fighting strength of regiments might be maintained in its efficiency. The necessary sacrifice of women involved in this point of view brought forth no protests, even from women, until the women of England were aroused to it by an attempt made to force the continental system upon that country.

THE CONTAGIOUS DISEASES ACTS. Early in the 19th century the military hierarchy had been desirous of establishing a regulated system in England, but the time did not seem propitious until well along in the mid-century, when the purpose crystallised.

A woman sounded the first warning. Harriet Martineau, with her finger always on the political pulse, foresaw the coming danger, and wrote several powerful letters of protest to the *Daily News* in 1859. In 1860 a Committee of the House of Lords sat to consider the advisability of introducing compulsory acts into India. Miss Martineau, in her autobiography, says that Florence Nightingale was called to give her opinion, and spoke strongly, with positive testimony against it. Nevertheless, between 1864 and 1869, the system was established in Great Britain by a series of Acts of Parliament passed with such haste and

Control of Prostitution 69

secrecy that, as is authoritatively stated in many published sources of reference, only about one tenth of the members knew of them. Introduced in late night sessions and rushed through with surreptitious haste, the first and second were only entering wedges, but the third established the full programme of regulation for all garrison towns and within a radius of fifteen miles around each one.

The first to give publicity to the new legislation, which was enforced with great secrecy, was the head of a Home for Girls, Daniel Cooper, who first suspected the onset of something new and menacing, and finally succeeded in obtaining a copy of the Acts. He exposed their iniquity, and was supported by two physicians, Dr. Charles Bell Taylor and Dr. Worth, who denounced them vigorously. But no headway was made in opposing them until all the moral forces of England were finally united under the leadership of Mrs. Josephine E. Butler,—one of the rare characters of the world, a perfect example of the exalted and fearless type of ideal womanhood;—one whose maternal protectiveness extended to every young and helpless creature.

SCOPE OF THE ACTS. The Acts empowered policemen in plain clothes, acting as spies, to arrest any woman in the territory covered by the law. The police were only obliged to "declare" that they "had reason for believing" the women to be immoral; it was therefore impossible to punish them for arresting innocent women, nor could informers be punished. Women thus arrested were requested to sign a paper called a "voluntary submission" (and ignorant ones were easily coerced into it) promising to present themselves at the periods ordered for medical examination, and, as an alternative, they had to defend their reputations in court. If they refused to submit to the medical examination, they could be sent to prison for disobedience. If, when examined, they were found to be diseased, they were committed to a hospital prison for compulsory treatment. If resistant, they were taken there by the police, and if they left it before being discharged they were liable to imprisonment with hard labour for one or two months. Under such a law, as an English writer pointed out, the police spies, acting on hints given them by persons acting in jealousy or revenge, or from motives of blackmail, "held the honour and reputation of every woman among the poorer classes absolutely at their disposal."

MRS. BUTLER'S CRUSADE. The women of England, united under Mrs. Butler's leadership in a national association, issued a declaration that the law was an insult and an outrage to every woman in the land, and protested against it on the following grounds: That laws are bound to define offences punishable by law. (No definition of prostitution was given in the Acts. It is indeed most difficult to define it technically and legally, and this difficulty has given rise to active controversy in every country where regulation has been in force.) That it was unjust to punish women only, and that the forced medical examinations were degrading punishments. That the Acts made it easier for young men to be impure. That the measures of enforcement were brutalising to all who took part in them. That venereal diseases had never been extirpated by such means, because their causes were moral and must be met by moral prevention. That to examine, treat, and isolate women only, while allowing infected men to go free, was a farce.

But a still higher ground was taken. Mrs. Butler insisted, in her speeches and writings, that the abolition movement was not merely a sex revolt, but was based on the conviction that impurity was as perilous for men as for women. It was as citizens first, and as women secondly, that they were in conflict with legislation that practically created a slave class. In her book, *The Constitution Violated*, Mrs. Butler defined clearly the

LEGAL AND CIVIC WRONGS OF REGULATION.

I. The first principle of jurisprudence in enlightened countries is that a suspected or accused person is protected against self-incrimination. The "voluntary submission" is a self-incrimination.

II. Enlightened countries hold an accused person innocent until he is proven guilty and so declared by a jury, but under the Contagious Diseases Acts the woman was held guilty until she could prove her innocence.

III. Constitutional law forbids indecent assault upon the person. The compulsory medical examination constituted an indecent assault.

Mrs. Butler showed further that the spy system necessitated by these laws subjected women to the arbitrary power of the police and removed them from the protection of the common law, and she made plain the inevitable confusion of the pub-

Control of Prostitution 73

lic conscience arising from the scruples of those persons who believe that the only wrong thing is disobedience to police regulations.

The protest embodying these civic and moral declarations is a historic human document which will be looked back upon with more and more veneration as the centuries pass. It was the first formal declaration of the revolt of women against the slavery of prostitution. It appeared in the *Daily News* on New Year's day, 1870, and was signed by two hundred and fifty of the great moral leaders among Englishwomen. Beginning with Harriet Martineau, there are many names known to literature, social reform, and advanced movements, and all the active suffragists of that day are enrolled there. Half-way down the column appears the name of Florence Nightingale.

THE STRUGGLE AGAINST THE ACTS. A long, desperate, and unremitting struggle followed the women's protest. Of three hundred prominent men in all walks of life, secular and religious, to whom, as an initial measure, Mrs. Butler first wrote letters of appeal for moral support, scarcely half a dozen gave a word of encouragement, while a group of aristocratic women signed a paper upholding the Acts. Mrs. Butler then turned for help to the public, and wrote her "Appeal to the People" in 1870. Tens of thousands of the working classes and plain people came to her support. Theirs were the daughters who were chiefly endangered.

Perhaps no other one woman has been more vilified or more venomously assailed by all the corrupt forces of society than was she. In several instances she narrowly escaped death from mob violence.

The contest was carried on for twelve years, and the abolition party grew to a membership of 50,000, but during all this time the Liberal party, with the great Mr. Gladstone at its head, resisted all appeals and ignored or belittled all testimony making for repeal of the Acts.

PROGRESS OF THE CRUSADE. In 1871, a Royal Commission recommended abolishing the compulsory examination, and raising the legal age of protection for girls from twelve years (as it then was) to fourteen. The first recommendation was not enacted into law until 1883. The second received some attention. The age of protection for little girls was with difficulty raised to thirteen, but not until 1885 was it possible to raise it to sixteen, so tenacious and determined was the resistance made to this amendment by the lawmakers of the nation. As late as 1880, two members of Parliament spoke on the floor of the House in favour of reducing the age of protection for little girls to below twelve years.

In 1880, '81, and '82, a Select Committee was appointed to inquire into the whole question of the workings of the Acts, and a number of women were called to testify. Among them was Mrs. Butler, whose evidence was very full, drawn entirely from personal knowledge, and couched in language of great, often exalted beauty; of moving and stirring power.

This Committee, in its report, endorsed the Acts, but did not recommend their extension, and it was felt that this was a victory. In 1881, and '82, there was also a Select Committee of the House of Lords on the white slave traffic, and in 1885 the *Pall Mall Gazette* published revelations of so shocking a nature regarding the trade that Parliament, until then most reluctant to act, was driven to pass some protective legislation. The odious Acts were repealed. They still, however, continue in force as to some of their main features in distant subjected provinces of the Empire under the guise of "rules."

RALLY OF THE REGULATIONISTS. During the progress of the women's crusade the upholders of regulation in all countries had been gathering re-enforcements and trying to strengthen their position. Government officials, military authorities, and even physicians reasserted the right of men to enslave and destroy women for their sensual pleasure. The *Lancet* upheld the registration of prostitutes. At an International Medical Congress in Vienna in 1873, strong resolutions were passed urging a convention of all nations and international agreements to establish the compulsory system of supervision of women in all the great seaport cities of the world.

On that occasion one member present said: "*From the moment when prostitution shall become a regular and recognised institution, admitted and regulated by the state, its perfect organisation will become possible.*" Another made an even more astounding proposition based upon the inoculation theory. Resolutions were framed calling upon England to summon a congress to form an international league for the regulation of

Control of Prostitution

prostitution. Dr. Collingwood, an English physician, protested nobly against this proposition, and Mrs. Butler and her allies, alarmed by the rising tide of domination of the regulationists, determined to organise an international movement in opposition to them. Mrs. Butler therefore undertook a continental tour in 1874, the year of the deepest discouragement and when everything looked darkest for the cause she had at heart. As a result of her travels and speeches the foes of vice in every country united into a powerful federation.

THE ABOLITIONIST CONGRESS AT GENEVA. In 1877 this body, the International Federation for the Abolition of State Regulation of Vice, as it is now called, met at Geneva, five hundred strong and representing seventeen countries, and passed a notable series of resolutions under the sections into which the congress was organised.

SECTION ON HYGIENE. It was resolved (briefly stated) that self-control in the relation between the sexes is one of the indispensable bases of the health of the individual and the community:— that prostitution is a fundamental violation of the laws of health; that the true function of public hygiene is not only to supervise disease, but to do all that makes for public health, which is, in its highest expression, inseparable from public morality:—that all systems of "Morals Police" were complete failures and the medical examination revolting to human nature and worthless as a sanitary measure by reason of its inevitable incompleteness; that it was impossible for the most serious forms of venereal disease to be so discovered or prevented and that it gave a false guarantee of the health of the women subjected to it.

SECTION ON MORALITY. Resolved that license is as reprehensible in men as in women:—that the regulation of prostitution destroys the idea of the unity of the moral law:—that in regulating vice the state forgets its duty to afford protection equally to both sexes, degrades women and incites youth to evil:—that the system of licensed houses raises prostitution to the rank of a profession and sanctions the immoral doctrine that debauch is a necessity for men.

SECTION ON SOCIAL ECONOMY. Exposed the whole condition of the economic dependency of women, and traced it to the inequality established by law between men and women, pointing to the unequal wages and sex slavery of women as proofs of their charges.

SECTION ON LEGISLATION. Resolved that the regulation of prostitution lowered women to the grade of chattels, putting them beyond the pale of the law and inducing the state to violate its own penal code and forget its duty of giving protection to the young.

DECLINE OF MEDICAL SUPPORT OF REGULATION. The congress of 1874 seemed to mark the highest point of medical advocacy of regulation, and at the medical congresses of 1876 and 1877 the subject was not allowed to come up, as it became known that fearless and determined antagonists would appear. At a Regulationist congress in 1894, only three supporters of the "Morals Police" were present.

It would be interesting and useful to know just how much of the change in the medical attitude has been due to the influence of women physicians. From the time of the entrance of the heroic Elizabeth Blackwell and her sister Emily

Hygiene and Morality

into this hitherto conservative profession, such women have consistently and steadily presented the nobler and more ethical—more spiritual—aspect of the questions relating to sex physiology and hygiene. Elizabeth Blackwell early declared, in a letter to her sister, her determination not to be intimidated or discouraged in the difficult task of attacking the social evil by methods of education, and her books and addresses on this subject are classics in their dignity and nobility of position. She was the first to address herself to parents. In 1852 she wrote to them of the Laws of Life in relation to girls, and in 1880 she wrote to them: "The fact must be clearly perceived and accepted that male chastity is a fundamental virtue in a State; that it secures the chastity of women, on which the moral qualities of fidelity, humanity, and trust depend, and that it secures the strength and truth of men, on which the intellectual vigour and wise government of a state depend."

From that time on women physicians as an entire body have stood unitedly for a single standard of morals and for the education of the public. In their ranks there can be found no division or opposing opinions on this subject. They are active in the warfare against vice, in every country

Control of Prostitution 81

where medicine has opened its doors to women, and, in our own country, they have been publicly called upon by their colleagues in the medical profession to carry the teachings of hygiene to the women of the land. Such women as Mary Putnam Jacobi, Sarah Hackett Stevenson, and Annie Daniels have brought medical science into perfect harmony with the most advanced civic standards, and their influence will be lasting.

THE FIRST AND SECOND CONFERENCES FOR THE PROPHYLAXIS OF SYPHILIS AND THE VENEREAL DISEASES. In 1899, the first international conference of important medical men and laymen met under this name in Brussels, and the second conference followed in the same city in 1902. An English writer says of the proceedings of these two weighty bodies that they marked the reconciliation of justice and morals with science.

The first conference took up six questions for discussion; they were: I. Systems of regulation now in force;—have they an influence on the frequency and the dissemination of syphilis and other venereal diseases? II. Medical supervision of prostitution;—is it capable of improvement? III. Tolerated houses;—is there, from the strictly medical point of view, any advantage in maintaining them, or is it better to suppress them? IV. Police supervision;—how to improve it. V. Number of women entering upon a life of prostitution;—how to decrease it. VI. What general propaganda could be made against prostitution?

Although much difference of opinion as to "regulation and control" was found to exist, as the discussions went on the following conclusions shaped themselves and were generally admitted.

1. The intervention of public powers in regulation as it exists has not given results of a certain or sufficient efficacy.

2. The prostitution of minor girls is most dangerous and should be the object of the most radical measures.

3. Better university instruction in venereology is needed.

4. The public power should be used to teach and to disseminate a knowledge of prostitution.

5. There should be a uniform system of statistics of prostitution and venereal diseases for all countries.

Disregarding all points on which there was

Control of Prostitution 83

an absence of unanimity, the conference passed a set of eight resolutions which were, in brief, as follows:

RESOLUTIONS OF THE FIRST BRUSSELS CONFERENCE. 1. All governments shall be called upon to suppress absolutely prostitution among minors. 2. Societies of Sanitary and Moral Prophylaxis should be formed in every country. 3. It is the duty of governments to promote, by complete and compulsory university courses, the instruction of truly competent medical specialists in venereal diseases. 4. Moral teaching should be provided for orphans. 5. The utmost rigour of the law should be applied to men who live upon the profits of prostitution (cadets, *souteneurs*, etc.). 6. Each country should appoint a commission to study conditions, investigate the number of hospital beds, dispensaries, and other opportunities for free treatment that are available. 7. Education in sex morality should be offered to the public. 8. There should be a uniform method of statistics adopted in all countries alike, as a basis of correct data for the combat against venereal diseases.

THE SECOND BRUSSELS CONFERENCE. The

84 Hygiene and Morality

conference of 1902 discussed public prophylaxis under the following heads:

A.—As to prostitution—what legal measures are advisable? I. The general protection of minors of both sexes. II. The improvement of public medical relief, hospital dispensaries, etc. III. Contagion:—by midwives; in obstetrics generally; in shops and factories; by instruments; as arising in the management of employment agencies and intelligence offices; as related to the policing of hotels and lodgings.

B.—A penal code for the transmission of venereal disease; should one be adopted?

The subject of private prophylaxis was considered under the two following heads: I. How to teach the public and especially the young. II. How to improve the public medical service.

Statistics and special communications closed the sessions. This second conference and indeed both were very remarkable not only for the facts brought out, but also as showing, along with the rapidly advancing tendency of the best medical thought to think in unison with social moralists on this question, two things especially: one, the immense handicap of involuntary, unconscious sex dominance and egotism to men discussing these problems: the other, the conspicuous ignorance of many great medical specialists in matters of sociology. It is a mistake to suppose that an eminent authority in one line will be equally eminent as an authority in another. As a matter of fact, the general esteem and confidence proffered to the medical profession by the public has sometimes encouraged its members to believe that their pronouncements on social conditions are as final as their definitions of medical knowledge. This has been pointed out by various critics of the proceedings of the two conferences at Brussels.

Dr. Pileur, an advocate of regulation, admitted that the diversity of opinion on this point was so great as to amount to anarchy. He would allow adult women to practise prostitution with the agreement of three [men] commissioners, and would hold them to strict rules, punishing them for infraction thereof. In his plan no men are to be punished.

That was his theory: his facts are impressive. He urges the reduction of prostitution to an irreducible minimum, and believes that cutting off the minors will bring this about. He states that seventy-five per cent. of all prostitution begins before the age of twenty-one; further, that of these minor girls fifty per cent. are afflicted with venereal disease and twenty-five per cent. have syphilis. These figures, he holds, are understated and would be higher if investigation could be thorough and precise. He judges by the statistics of such girls as had been finally arrested in Paris as "clandestines," of whom seventy-two per cent. were found to be diseased when arrested. He holds that the prostitution of minors is the absolutely capital fact in the question of prostitution and insists that if all under twenty-one could be kept out, the number of women choosing the life, who might be called "chronic" or "persevering" prostitutes, would be surprisingly small. From a medical standpoint, he considers older women as less liable to disease, and estimates the amount of syphilis among them as seventeen per cent.

Dr. Neisser stated that the unanimous testimony of all nations was that irregular intercourse, especially that of prostitution, was the main source of all ravages by venereal diseases. The three factors in prostitution that are fatal in the hygienic sense are: Frequency of sex relations; absence of choice among persons; constant variety of persons. Prostitution is the knot around which contamination centres. Individual immoral relations are less dangerous, and, if infection then occurs, it has been accidentally introduced from prostitution. Nevertheless, he advocated the recognition and toleration of prostitution as a trade, unavoidable under present social conditions, and believes that it strengthens the control of the police over thieves and criminals to have the management of prostitution within their jurisdiction. After expounding this last-mentioned curious social view, he advocated teaching the principle of chastity to young men.

Henri Monod, an uncompromising abolitionist, quoted from many sources to show that real depravity is not a serious cause of prostitution. Few women find any enjoyment in this life. They regard it, not as pleasure, but as "work." M. Monod quoted some statistics of Dr. Le Pileur, to show the ages at which 582 girls were drawn into prostitution.

AGES AT WHICH GIRLS WERE RUINED:

6 were ruined when from 10–11 years old.
2 " " " " 11–12 " "
8 " " " " 12–13 " "
24 " " " " 13–14 " "

88 Hygiene and Morality

  50 were ruined when from 14–15 years old.
 142   " " " " 15–16 " "
 106   " " " " 16–17 " "
  86   " " " " 17–18 " "
  67   " " " " 18–19 " "
  38   " " " " 19–20 " "
  24   " " " " 20–21 " "
  11   " " " " 21–22 " "
  11   " " " " 22–23 " "
   3   " " " " 23–24 " "
   1 was " " " 24–25 " "
   3 were " " " 25–26 " "

[A set of figures corroborative of these, though not presented at the conference, are added here as being germane to the heading. They are given by the Rev. G. P. Merrick, in his *Work Among the Fallen*.

    11 ruined before 11 years of age.
    36   "   "   12 " " "
    62   "   "   13 " " "
   104   "   "   14 " " "
   358   "   "   15 " " "
 1,192   "   "   16 " " "
 1,425   "   "   17 " " "
 1,369   "   "   18 " " "
 1,158   "   "   20 " " "
   947   "   "   21 " " "
   703   "   "   22 " " "

He also makes statements that agree with those

of M. Monod, viz., that out of 100,000 cases personally known to him he had not found one hundred who did not loathe the life. Drink, said he, was a necessity to nerve them to endure it.]

Certain ones of the members of the conference of 1902 advocated laws making the transmission of venereal disease a penal offence. The weak points of this proposal were forcibly presented by Miss Blanche Leffingwell, of England, who pointed out: I. Danger of unjust accusation; II. Opportunities for blackmail; III. Dangers of publicity; IV. Avoidance of such retaliation by the self-respecting and its exploitation by the vile; V. Resultant estrangement of patients from physicians; VI. Resultant fostering of quackery.

Careful reading of the full proceedings leaves the settled conviction that the advocates of toleration and regulation have a weak case, contradict themselves and one another, and grasp wildly at the most absurd social remedies; while the abolitionists are logical, rational, unanimous, and show some knowledge of human nature and of social conditions. Again avoiding all controversial themes, the second conference agreed unanimously on the following resolutions: That there should be full, adequate, free hospital treat-

90   Hygiene and Morality

ment for all cases of venereal disease; that patients should not be regarded as guilty persons, but simply as patients; that teaching in sex hygiene should be given to soldiers; that the education of the public should be continued and that emphasis should be laid on the doctrine that the health of young men is improved by continence; that uniform statistics should be kept; that the physiology of sex should be taught in the schools of all countries to the children of all ages. This done, the conference adjourned without fixing a date for reassembling, leaving the societies that had been formed at its instigation to carry on the work in their own countries.

THE SOCIETIES OF SANITARY AND MORAL PROPHYLAXIS. Among these national societies newly formed to carry on educational missions in regard to venereal diseases, the American Society of Sanitary and Moral Prophylaxis, under the presidency of its founder, Dr. Prince A. Morrow of New York City, stands easily in the lead by reason of its singleness of purpose (certain others still wrestling with the vexed question of regulation), the unassailable dignity of its tone in promulgating a teaching which harmonises the soundest medical science with a high morality, and its resultant widespread influence. Its membership is open to men and women, to the professions and to the laity, and this association, as well as the State Societies to which it has given the impulse, offers the needed opportunity for all who desire to ally themselves with the new crusade for the attainment of the single moral standard and the extirpation of the diseases of immorality.

REGULATION PASSING FROM THE CONTINENT. The reports of the Brussels Conference show that regulation is being discredited in the countries where it has long been under trial. Norway abolished the Morals Police in 1888, and since then the Norwegian women have defeated provisions that they believed portended a return to regulation.

Denmark and Sweden both reported a probable early cessation of police control with retention of medical inspection only. Italy has abolished regulation.

France has had two government commissions studying the subject; one, appointed in 1901, had no results. The second, appointed in 1903, upon which one woman was placed, gave a verdict of banishment for regulation; decided that prostitution is not a legal offence coming under the penal law, but is a social phenomenon to be combated, but not with force; agreed that it should be made punishable to "procure" even adults, even with their own consent, and framed a number of resolutions looking to a rational and humane discouragement of prostitution as a business, as well as to the treatment of venereal diseases. Their conclusions have not yet been enacted into legislation, but the force of public opinion will probably soon prevail over the small group of determined regulationists who still resist them.

DANGER OF REGULATION NOT PAST. In spite of all the available testimony against it, tolerated and licensed vice still finds advocates. Arguments in its favour have been advanced, and efforts made to introduce regulation systems in this country. Doubtless such efforts will be repeated, from time to time, and it is therefore most important that the moral public should be well grounded in the lessons taught by English and continental experience, and ready to make intelligent resistance to any such attempted invasion.[1]

[1] See Appendix A.

There have always been, and perhaps always will be, some honest and well-intentioned apologists for regulation. The existing writings and speeches made by members of this class, however, such as may be found in the transactions of a society organised in England during the crusade against the Contagious Diseases Acts, whose aim was to support regulation, show, alongside of perfectly good intentions, an extreme mediocrity of intelligence, a very limited point of view, and a profound ignorance of their subject. Such banal opinions as that erring girls would find, in the police, wise and benevolent friends, who would lead them back to their families; and that inscribed women would become so accustomed to the routine of their supervised lives as to miss it if discontinued, show sufficiently the worth of their information.

On the other hand, all accounts teem with evidence of the disastrous results of regulatory legislation, and this evidence will now be summed up, at the risk of a certain amount of repetition, in order to bring all the arguments of the opposition into one place.

BRUTALISING EFFECT OF REGULATION ON

CHARACTER. A terrible revelation is that of the brutalising effect of regulatory enactments upon the natures of those who administer and enforce them. This was strikingly shown in all the evidence laid before the Select Committee in England, and appears again in the reports of the Brussels conferences. Officers of the army and military surgeons were seen to have reverted to the brute; as in the case of the one who ordered an establishment for his regiment in advance, and, knowing well that many would be little girls, excused this on the ground that "In India prostitution begins in the cradle": and of the other, who granted permits for licensed houses. A menacing disregard for the good of the civil community was suggested in the testimony of such men, that "diseased women, if incurable, were expelled from the cantonment." But, it was asked,—where did they go? For, unless they could die at once, they must go somewhere and be a danger to their environment.

Equally disturbing evidence of the decline of traditional chivalry under the effects of the supervision of vice is at hand in the suggestion of a German surgeon, who, angered by the failure of inscribed women to appear regularly for examination, would have had them whipped for absence; and in that of a French doctor who proposed imprisoning each woman for several days before examination, in order to prevent their tampering with symptoms. The quarrels and disputes between medical and police supervisors have also been numerous and undignified.

In reading such material, one feels keenly that the supervision of vice degrades the medical profession to a plane little higher than that of the cadet or *souteneur*.

THE INSULT TO RELIGION. The insult to religion was deadly. There was (and still is) a wide-spread belief in distant provinces that licensed prostitution was a part of the Christian religion. The editor of *The Sentinel* pointed out the incongruity of ordinances passed "in the year of our LORD" for licensing vice, and Mrs. Butler, in her evidence, said, "Few things shock the sense of the country more than the fact that religious teaching is allied with state regulation of vice." Even as late as 1908 the statement appeared in an English journal that one reason for an outbreak of syphilis in an African province was "the introduction of Christianity."

THE SANITARY INEFFICIENCY OF REGULATION. The entire mass of testimony makes it clear that state regulation, licensing, and medical examination does not diminish venereal disease. Conflicting and contradictory columns of statistics do not alter this conclusion. Dr. Mounier of Utrecht says that statistical methods are futile in the clearing up of disputes as to the efficacy of regulation. Figures showing results favourable to regulation were based on imperfect knowledge. One prominent error, made before the discovery of the *Spirochæte pallida*, was in the confusing of venereal ulcer with syphilis. The difference between them was not understood. Remembering that venereal ulcer is the least serious and most readily cured of the venereal diseases, it will at once be clear that its figures might easily show an improvement which, if credited to the graver disease, would be most misleading. Again, remembering the variable period of inoculation of the *Spirochæte pallida*, and the latency of the *gonococcus*, possibilities of error are evidently many. Still another source of error lay here: it has been found that syphilis shows a certain variability when observed over long periods of time, having its epochs of increase and decrease.

This obscure and, to many, unknown phenomenon makes observations over short time-periods of little value.

The reasons for the sanitary failure of regulation may be tabulated as follows:

I. THE ONE-SIDED EXAMINATION. It is surprising that the plan of examining women only while men were unexamined should ever have been advanced as worthy of being taken seriously. Morrow says of this: "The prostitute is but the purveyor of the infection;—she simply returns to her male partner, the prostituant, as he is called, the infection which she has received from another prostituant. In the ultimate analysis it will be found that the male is the chief malefactor." Again he says: "The health officer of a port might as well attempt to prevent the importation of infectious disease from a plague-infested vessel by quarantining the infected women while permitting the infected men to go free." This weakness has been admitted in official circles, and Neisser and others at the conference of 1902 advocated examining every man who entered a house of ill-fame. The naïveté of this suggestion speaks for itself. Men would not submit to it. This precaution has been tried occasionally in armies and navies and has been rejected as a "degradation" involving "loss of respect" to the men.

II. LENGTH OF TIME BETWEEN EXAMINATIONS. The usual time of one or two weeks between examinations is too long. A woman may appear free from disease at one time and develop an infectious discharge before the next. This has also been recognised and more frequent examination recommended—even one or two weekly. But aside from the great expense to the taxpayers (many of whom are women) in supporting a staff large enough to make this everywhere possible, it is acknowledged that even the most enslaved women would rebel.

III. MEDIATE CONTAGION. Mechanical transmission of disease or "mediate contagion" is believed to be possible. The woman in this case, remaining uninfected herself, passes on to one man an infection which she has received from another.

IV. CLANDESTINE PROSTITUTION. The difficulty of the "clandestine" is perhaps the most obstinate of all. So great is the detestation of police and medical control among women that the greatest zeal and energy on the part of the officials cannot prevent numbers of them from practising secretly. While all medical authorities agree that these are the most dangerous prostitutes, the most unfaltering believers in regulation can give no suggestion for strengthening this weak link in the chain. This weakness has been realised in every country where regulation has been tried. Pontoppidan wrote in 1903 that 5000 women were inscribed by the police of Paris, in that year, while there were 50,000 clandestines. Figures for Berlin in 1896 were even worse; viz., 4039 women inscribed, while the number of clandestines equalled that of Paris. Dr. Käthe Schirmacher has recently stated that the police of Paris, in the last thirty years, had arrested 725,000 women and had inscribed 155,000. Twenty-five per cent. of those inscribed, she added, had disappeared.

V. REGULATION INCREASES VICE. Ample testimony is at hand to show that immoral practices increase with the sense of security imparted by official inspection. In the words of Dr. C. Bell Taylor, there is "multiplied indulgence springing from the apparent immunity." In armies it has been understood that the government purposed providing the regiments with "clean girls," and in civil communities young men speak openly of the advantages of licensed houses. The more wide-spread immoral practices are, the greater of course must be the danger of infection.

VI. IGNOMINY ATTACHES TO TREATMENT. Under regulation the ignominy attaching to the compulsory treatment deters respectable patients from seeking medical aid; brings the special hospital into disrepute and fosters the industry of quacks, who offer secrecy and regard for the sensitive pride of the individual. The seriousness of this danger is widely recognised.

Pontoppidan, after a moderate and rational review of the whole subject, says: "Control is entirely without positive value as a security."

IMMORAL NATURE OF REGULATION. Aside from sanitary inefficiency, regulation stands condemned on the following counts:

1. It corrupts and demoralises the police and offers endless opportunities for blackmail and extortion. Here it may be emphasised that, although there is in the United States no

Control of Prostitution

legal regulation of vice, yet there is blackmail and extortion because the police, under the pressure of corrupt social elements have developed a system of protection for vice which approaches closely to an official alliance with it.

2. It exposes innocent women to persecution. Numerous instances of this kind are on record. Respectable girls have been reported to the police from motives of revenge or jealousy, and self-supporting women have been driven from positions and their property manipulated away from them. Cases have been known where such victims have been driven to suicide.

3. That it perpetuates a class of women who are deprived of the protection of the law has been referred to. For such women, no matter what their just grievance, justice in the courts would be a thing unheard of. Even without regulation it is doubtful whether legal justice exists for these unfortunates.

4. Regulation bears with special hardship on the poorest women. Indeed, it may be said that only the very poor and defenceless are exposed to its full horrors. The fact that immoral women who are able to command ample means are safe against the severities of the law has been

frequently mentioned by writers belonging to different countries.

5. It puts governments in the position of endorsing the assumption that women may be sacrificed for men's pleasure. It even tends to make it appear that women are the chief offenders and the primary corrupting influence, and may therefore be treated with a disregard of justice and decency. On this point M. Jules Favre said: "The worst that could befall the public health is nothing to the corruption of morals and national life engendered, propagated, and prolonged by the system of official surveillance." Again, with regulation, the state is placed in a position not clearly different from that of the individual agents of immorality, and all taxpayers, women as well as men, are compelled to pay for the maintenance of officials to supervise prostitution. A German member of the Reichstag, speaking on this point, said: "The state which officially tolerates and guarantees houses of prostitution assumes the rôle of Procurer, a delinquent whom the German penal code punishes with imprisonment and hard labour."

6. It destroys respect for women and thus tends to make men unmanly and cowardly. And

the flourishing and unrestricted commercial prostitution which has been permitted to develop in the United States breeds this same contempt and unmanliness.

7. It blights that high ideal of parenthood and especially of motherhood that consecrates the functions of physical life. And the very existence of prostitution, regulated or unregulated, brings on this blight. No one has dwelt upon this truth more earnestly than Mrs. Butler. In her testimony before the Commons Committee she said:

> There is nothing in the physical being of a man that corresponds to the sacredness of the maternal functions in a woman, and these functions, and every organ connected with them, ought to be held in reverence by man. When this reverence ceases to be felt through the habitual outrage of any class of women, however degraded that class may already be, the demoralisation of society at large is sure to follow.

8. Finally, it is clear that the various systems of police protection and state licensing of prostitution have been the breeder and the main security of the most shocking of modern evils, the white slave traffic.

Systems of "segregation" deserve the same condemnation as regulation and for the same reasons.

CHAPTER II

THE WHITE SLAVE TRAFFIC

THAT this trade in girls for immoral purposes has grown naturally and inevitably out of the continental system of regulated vice is too evident to be contested. The existence of this traffic was at first undreamed of by Mrs. Butler and her associates, but they soon came into collision with it. In 1879, the Rev. Mr. Dyer received information that a young English girl was detained against her will in a licensed house in Brussels, and intended committing suicide as the only escape. By the aid of a Belgian clergyman she was rescued, and then began a life and death struggle for the exposure of the evil. In time the British Society succeeded in obtaining the names of many men and women who were systematically engaged in this trade in London, as well as the addresses of fifty licensed houses in France, Belgium, and Holland, to which the girls were sold. They also succeeded in

The White Slave Traffic

exposing all the methods and practices in the trade. It was shown that the exculpatory statements of the police were false in every particular; that girls were decoyed under pretence of obtaining employment, and that there were systematic methods of intimidation. It was proved that girls were asked in foreign tongues whether they came willingly, and then, not understanding, or thinking they were entering domestic service, they were inscribed as having come of their own free will. Again, they were listed under false names and then threatened with imprisonment for "forgery" if they rebelled. All street clothes were taken from them. A skilful system involved them deeply in debt to their captors. If resistant, they were beaten and starved. Padded cells were found in the houses which were visited daily by the police, even the windows and doors being covered. It was also shown that the names, persons, and pursuits of the foreign agents in England were perfectly well known to the police and had been so for years, but "the state of the English law did not authorise" their arrest or extradition. As investigations went deeper the traffic in England was traced back to the year 1857.

The experience gained in this crusade led Mrs. Butler to say:

> As an inevitable and necessary accompaniment of the establishment of licensed houses of prostitution under government patronage all over the world, there exists the most extensive slave traffic in the interests of vice. This fact has become . . . fully acknowledged during the last few years.

In a memorandum to the Committee of the House of Lords M. de Laveleye wrote:

> The white slave traffic is carried on . . . and will not be suppressed as long as prostitution constitutes, on the continent, a traffic, not only tolerated but legalised, privileged, and licensed in the same way as any other traffic. The legal organisation of debauchery is the chief support of the odious trade against which we are seeking a remedy. . . . This state of things, which places prostitution on the footing of a recognised commerce, must naturally produce a most dire effect on the police and on all who are brought into contact with these abominable institutions. . . . The traffic in women, that is to say, the letting on hire of human beings for debauchery, as of horses and other cattle, is a system contrary to all morality and all sense of right and ought to be universally forbidden. As long as these establishments remain legalised institutions, the traffic which supplies them will not be stopped.

THE SHARE OF LAW IN THE WHITE SLAVE

The White Slave Traffic

TRAFFIC. The members of the British Society were not long in discovering how much the laws of the country had to do with the extent and the security of the trade in girls. Briefly stated, the features of the laws relating to the protection of girls were, at that time, as follows: To abduct a girl under twenty-one for immoral purposes was a felony, if she belonged to a propertied class or family. If she was propertyless, it was only a misdemeanour to abduct her under sixteen. Thus a penniless girl, sixteen years old, could be lawfully decoyed for immoral purposes, as she could claim no protection from the state or its agents the police. (And here again let it be recalled that women wage-earners and women taxpayers were helping to provide the public funds needed for maintaining such legislation.) But still worse was the discovery that girls having neither parents nor guardians might safely be abducted even under sixteen, as the law provided no penalty at all for such act, nor any protection for such girls. Here was obviously a deliberate and intentional legal omission devised by legislators with the sole and single purpose of maintaining a supply of victims,—not, perhaps, for the white slave trade, but for the institution of prostitution.

This cannot be too plainly stated. Such careful legal fencing could not be accidental; and that it was indeed not accidental was fully proved, later, by the long and stubborn resistance of the lawmakers to any amendment.

Another strange feature of these strangely unchivalrous laws, was that a father, having reason to believe, but not possessing legal proof, that his daughter was in a house of prostitution, could not secure a search-warrant to look for her, nor could any benevolent friend do so.

FACTS LEARNED OF THE TRADE IN GIRLS. The following facts were brought out as to the trade in girls: girls between sixteen and twenty were the most desirable, because the most docile.

It was important to entrap only healthy girls, as, if any were found to be diseased and to require hospital care, the trade lost money.

A skilled system of falsehood was practised in order to evade the fairly strict laws of continental countries relating to minors.

The police were always in sympathy and sometimes in guilty complicity with the agents and the tolerated houses. One European police official explained their attitude thus: "We cannot

The White Slave Traffic

injure establishments legally authorised and in which so much capital is vested." The English committee declared: "Reliance on the police has misled all who have trusted to it."

Intelligence offices, all licensed, were the main avenues of the trade. The girls were called "colis" (packages) and the business was perfectly organised, with routes, ports, agents, and travellers; cargoes and technical phraseology, prices and values all worked out.

English birth certificates (false) were bought for a small sum.

Four fifths of the girls so enslaved were orphans.

A close relation was found to exist between the city authorities and keepers or owners of tolerated houses. The first exposure in Brussels implicated the mayor and two aldermen, all of whom resigned.

THE STRUGGLE FOR IMPROVED LEGISLATION. The history of the attempts made to amend these laws is highly instructive, as showing the different points of view of the governed and the governing, and the opposition of interests between enfranchised men and unenfranchised women.

The Society sent a memorial to the proper minister in 1880 asking for a deputation to be received. A year went by without answer. On making a second appeal, the committee were informed that official inquiry had been made and it had been found that the Society had overstated the case. A petition signed by 1000 women was then presented by Mrs. Butler in 1881. An inquiry by the House of Lords followed. Two years later the Lords reported, making various recommendations for the better protection of girls. The House of Lords passed these measures, and the House of Commons defeated them. The same thing was repeated in 1884. In 1885 a third bill, in which the "age of consent" was set at fifteen years, was about to be killed in the House of Commons, when the *Pall Mall Gazette*[1] brought out its revelations which aroused the public wrath and drove the legislators to act.

THE WHITE SLAVE TRAFFIC IN THE UNITED STATES. As the revelations of the international traffic in young girls were unfolded, leaders of communities formed National Vigilance Leagues to carry on a war of extermination against it. There are now Leagues in Great Britain, Germany, France, Russia, Sweden, Norway, Belgium, Hol-

[1] July 10, 1885.

land, Italy, Spain, Portugal, Switzerland, Austria, and the United States, the latter having been formed in 1906 with O. Edward Janney, M.D., of Baltimore, as its president. These Leagues have brought about an international agreement by which the governments of the countries represented bind themselves to a concerted action in suppression of the white slave trade. In 1907, Congress passed an act designed to crush the traffic in foreign girls, as the limitations of the constitution of the United States confine its jurisdiction to immigrants. This act provided that any person who should keep, maintain, support, or harbour any alien woman for immoral purposes within three years after her arrival in this country should be punishable for misdemeanour by five years' imprisonment or $5000 fine. The federal government has no power over traffic in American women, carried on within the States themselves.

In the process of enforcing the law regarding aliens the United States District Attorney at Chicago was directed to take the proper steps for securing the conviction of certain persons who were suspected of violating the statute. The raids upon houses of prostitution and arrests of their inmates that were made with this end in view brought to light a mass of evidence of a terrible, much of an unspeakable nature, and the District Attorney, Edwin W. Sims, and his assistant, H. D. Parkin, as well as convicting a number of procurers, felt it their duty to make known to American parents the conditions imperilling their daughters, as it was evident that a profound state of ignorance prevailed as to the existence in our country of so vile a trade. They therefore wrote a series of articles for a popular magazine in which the facts they had learned were most clearly and explicitly stated. Their investigations led them to believe that some 65,000 American girls and 15,000 aliens are being entrapped yearly for the white slave trade. The methods by which they are taken vary: promises of employment, bogus messages, plausible invitations, deceptive marriage ceremonies, even real marriage. The runaway marriage is a device frequently used with country girls of American families. The District Attorney believed that there was a syndicate which carried on a business in the ruin of girls as steady, regular, and systematic as any great business of a legitimate kind, and that its ramifications extended to the Pacific with dis-

The White Slave Traffic

tributing centres in nearly all the large cities. Recent Congressional commissions of inquiry believe that no definite syndicate exists, but that there is a general understanding between the agents in different cities. This is, of course, equally menacing and serious, and does not relieve the situation of its darkness.

Of the details of the life, Sims repeats almost the very words of the English investigators into the Brussels conditions. He writes:

When a white slave is sold and landed in a house or dive she becomes a prisoner . . . in each of these places is a room having but one door, to which the keeper holds the key. Here are locked all the street clothes, shoes, and ordinary apparel . . . the finery provided for the girls is of a nature to make their appearance on the street impossible. Then, in addition to this handicap, the girl is placed at once in debt to the keeper for a wardrobe . . . she cannot escape while she is in debt, and she can never get out of debt. . . . Not many of the women in this class expect to live more than ten years—perhaps the average is less. Many die painful deaths by disease [venereal] many by consumption, but it is hardly beyond the truth to say that suicide is their general expectation. . . . The facts that I have stated are for the awakening of parents and guardians of girls.

Among the individual instances described by

the District Attorney was that of a little girl who was fourteen years old when stolen, and who, besides being used as a scrubwoman by day, in two and one half years' time had been compelled to earn eight thousand dollars for her owner.

The statement made at the Brussels conference, that the number of chronic or persevering prostitutes, if separated from the others, would be surprisingly small, is borne out by Sims's declaration that only about twenty per cent. of all prostitutes are willingly such, or have chosen or preferred the life, while all the other eighty per cent. have either been forced into it by poverty and destitution, or have been betrayed, trapped, enticed, or sold into it.

The National Vigilance League has published a pamphlet called *The Nation and the Traffic in Women*, addressed to the American people, in which ample facts as to the present situation are set forth with moderation and as entire absence of sensationalism as the extraordinary truth permits.

The facts speak for themselves, and the ultimate responsibility for these conditions, in an unscrupulous use of property, and in the protection secured for vice by corrupt sordid elements of

The White Slave Traffic

society who have been permitted to seize the machinery of government for their own evil and mercenary purposes, is laid squarely where it belongs, at the doors of the business community and respectable citizens of the country.

Mention is made of a city "where the authorities seem to regard the slavery of young girls as a part of the legitimate business of the city." Of another, where the money to build slave pens was furnished by the business men of the town. Procurers of young girls, it is pointed out, "are useful to the politicians, and, when arrested, escape through political influence—while smart lawyers are employed to defend them when arrested."

The hopes of dealing an effectual blow to the white slave trade were painfully frustrated by the decision of the Supreme Court of the United States early in 1909, which set free the traders, accused by the federal authorities, on the ground of the unconstitutionality of that clause in the immigration law under which they were prosecuted. This leaves the future status of white slave traders to the slow and uncertain action of the legislatures of the States of the Union, many of which, it has been found, have failed

116   Hygiene and Morality

entirely to provide adequate protection for young girls.[1]

THE LAWS OF PROTECTION FOR GIRLS IN THE UNITED STATES. How high the standards of the States are likely to be may be conjectured from the provisions of those laws designed to give protection to girls, which are commonly known as the laws of the age of consent.

This age, beyond which there is no legal protection for girls against seduction and violation of the person, nor punishment for men committing such acts, was originally fixed by the common law at TEN YEARS.

No American State took any steps toward raising this age until 1864. From that time to the present, the insistent urging of women has brought about some gradual amendment, though, with the fixing of a higher age limit, the corresponding penalties have usually been reduced, and thirteen States name no penalty at all for violation of the law. The following data are taken from the *History of Woman Suffrage*, by Susan B. Anthony and Ida Husted Harper, and are there carried up

---

[1] The federal law of 1910 which, at the time of writing, is before Congress, has not had time to prove its effectiveness.

The White Slave Traffic

to the year 1900. It has been thought best to retain that year as a dividing line, and leave changes made since that time for mention in future revisions.

Three States then had the age of ten years fixed as the age of protection against rape. They were Florida, Georgia, and Mississippi. Florida, however, recognised two grades of protection: the age of consent (ten), and the age of protection (sixteen at first, later raised to eighteen). Certain details will be given on a subsequent page.

Two States, Kentucky and West Virginia, gave protection up to twelve years. One, New Hampshire, to thirteen years. Ten, Alabama, Illinois, Indiana, Maine, Missouri, Nevada, New Mexico, South Carolina, Virginia, Wisconsin, to fourteen years. Two, Iowa and Texas, to fifteen years. Nineteen, Arkansas, California, Connecticut, Dakota, District of Columbia, Louisiana, Maryland, Massachusetts, Michigan, Minnesota, Montana, New Jersey, Ohio, Oregon, Pennsylvania, Rhode Island, Tennessee, Vermont, Washington to sixteen years. Nine, Arizona, Colorado, Delaware, Idaho, Kansas, Nebraska, New York, Utah, Wyoming, to eighteen years.

Some brief account of the ways in which

Hygiene and Morality

amendments to these laws have been brought about will be instructive as showing that it is not easy to improve them.

Arkansas raised the protected age from twelve to sixteen in 1893. But the penalty, which had previously been not less than five years nor more than twenty-five, was reduced to one year.

In California the Women's Christian Temperance Union asked the legislature in 1887 to raise the protected age from ten (as it then was) to eighteen. The legislature raised it to fourteen. In 1895 the women secured an amendment fixing it at eighteen. The governor vetoed it. In 1897 the women tried again, and secured a bill fixing sixteen as the protected age; this was finally passed and became law.

Dakota raised the age from ten to fourteen in 1887. In 1895, the women of Dakota tried to obtain legislation fixing the age at eighteen, but only succeeded in getting sixteen years enacted into law. Moreover the penalty was lowered and the following clause introduced:

> No conviction can be had in case the female is over ten years and the man under the age of twenty and if it appears to the satisfaction of the jury that the female was sufficiently matured and informed to

understand the nature of the act and to consent thereto.

In Delaware the age of *seven years only* was legally protected against the brutality of man until 1889. In that year the women of the State petitioned the legislature and secured fifteen years, but the penalties were lowered and no minimum penalty was fixed. In 1895 the women brought another plea and obtained eighteen years. It is, however, very difficult to secure convictions and in cases where men have been convicted they have been pardoned.

In Florida, the women of the Christian Temperance Union made many attempts to have the age of consent and of protection both raised, from, respectively, ten and sixteen years to eighteen. Their bills were always laid on the table. In 1901, they made a valiant effort with two bills: the one, raising the age of protection against rape from ten to fourteen, passed the House but was lost in the Senate; the other, raising the age of protection from sixteen to eighteen, was finally forced through by a small majority and in the face of all manner of obstructive devices, but no minimum penalty was attached to it. The age

Hygiene and Morality

of protection against rape remained at ten years, with loopholes for the evasion of the penalty.

In Georgia, the suffrage association of Atlanta tried to raise the protected age from ten to eighteen. The bill was killed in committee. In 1899, the attempt was again made. The Women's Christian Temperance Union also came forward, asking for twenty-one years. A bill raising the age to twelve was brought in and defeated. Reconsidered at the plea of the women, it was redefeated more emphatically.

In Indiana, bills urged by women to raise the age above fourteen have never been permitted to come out of committee.

Iowa amended her law in 1886, raising the age from ten to thirteen. In 1896, the Women's Christian Temperance Union secured an advance to fifteen, with heavy penalty, but a clause provides that the man cannot be convicted on the testimony of the injured person without corroborative testimony.

In Kansas, immediately after women obtained municipal suffrage, the age of consent was raised from ten to eighteen years. The law of Colorado was also carried by the women's vote in their first year of exercising the franchise.

The White Slave Traffic

Michigan raised the age of consent from ten to fourteen in 1887. In 1895, an amendment to eighteen was introduced and passed, but the day after the friends of the bill, thinking it safe, had gone home, it was reconsidered and changed to sixteen.

Minnesota altered the age from ten to sixteen in 1891. Thousands of women had petitioned in vain for eighteen.

New York raised its protected age for girls in 1887 from ten years to sixteen. A few years later there was an attempt made to reduce it to twelve. The women made themselves heard in indignant protest and the effort was relinquished. In 1895 the age of eighteen was legally secured. It is, however, almost impossible to secure convictions and many flagrant cases of assault on little girls go unpunished, the writer's long experience as a district nurse having brought a number of such cases to her personal knowledge, where the miscreants have been sheltered behind political and police protection.

It is natural to wonder what arguments men can find for defending such standards on the floors of legislatures: this has been answered by Dr. Elizabeth Blackwell from English history, and

American records show the same reasons given. One is, the need of protecting men against blackmail for false charges, and the other, the physical fact of the early oncoming of puberty in little girls. That it is possible for a child of twelve to become pregnant has seemed to legislators of this type reason enough for regarding her as a matured woman.

SOURCES OF MATERIAL USED IN THE PREPARATION OF PART II

American Society of Moral and Sanitary Prophylaxis. Transactions. All volumes.
Ames, Sheldon, A Comparative Survey of Laws in Force for the Prohibition, Regulation, and Licensing of Vice in England and other Countries. London, 1877.
Blaschko, A., Syphilis und Prostitution vom Standpunkte der öffentlichen Gesundheitspflege. Berlin, 1893.
Booth, C., The Iniquity of State-Regulated Vice. London, 1884.
British Committee of the I. F. A. S. R. V. The Shield. London.
Brussels. Conférence Internationale pour le Prophylaxie de la Syphilis et des Maladies Venériennes. 1899.
——, The same. Second Conference, 1902.
Butler, Josephine E., A Grave Question. London, 1885 or 1886.
Butler, Josephine E., Personal Reminiscences of a Great Crusade. London, 1896.
Butler, Josephine E., Principles of the Abolitionists. London, 1885.
Butler, Josephine E., The Revival and Extension of the Abolitionist Cause. London, 1887.
Committee of Fifteen, The, The Social Evil, with Special Reference to New York. New York, 1902.
Congrès des Sciences Médicales, Compte Rendu Résumé, Troisième Session, Vienne, 1873. Paris, 1876.
Dolléans, E., La Police des Mœurs. Paris, 1903.
Dyer, A. S., The European Slave Trade. London, 1880.

Dyer, A. S., The Slave Trade in European Girls to India. London, 1893.
Fiaux, F. L., La Police des Mœurs. Paris, 1888.
Geneva. Conférence du Genève, 1899. Fédération Abolitioniste Internationale. Compte Rendu. Geneva, 1900.
Guyot, Yves. Prostitution under the Regulation System, 1884.
House of Commons, Select Committee to Inquire into the Contagious Diseases Acts. Report, 3 vols., 1880, 1881, 1882.
House of Commons, Select Committee on the Contagious Diseases Acts. Minority Report. Reprinted from Parliamentary Papers, 340, Session of 1882.
House of Lords Committee, Prostitution in Hong Kong. (Parliamentary Paper C. 309.)
House of Lords Committee on the Law Relating to the Protection of Young Girls. Report, 1881. Appendix.
House of Lords Committee on the Law Relating to the Protection of Young Girls. Reports and Papers. Vol. ix.
Joest, Wilhelm, Du Japon en Allemagne par le Sibéris. [Routes, ports, cargoes, etc., of white slave trade.]
Ladies' National Association for the Abolition of Government Regulation of Vice. Publications, London.
Ladies' National Association for the Repeal of the Contagious Diseases Acts, Reports, Liverpool, 1871. Tracts on the Contagious Diseases Acts, 1871, 1883.
London Committee for Suppressing the Traffic in British Girls. Reports 1881, 1885, 1886.
McClure, S. S., The Tammanyising of a Civilisation. In McClure's Magazine, November, 1909.
Martineau, Harriet, Autobiography. Edited by M. W. Chapman, London, 1877.
Martineau, Harriet, Letters on State Regulation of Vice. In Daily News, 1859.
Scheven, Katharina, Denkschrift über die in Deutschland bestehenden Verhältnisse in Bezug auf das Bordellwesen. In Schriften des Bundes Deutscher Frauenvereine, Heft. VI., 1904.
Schirmacher, Käthe, M.D., The Work of the Extra-Parlia-

Sources of Material Used 125

mentary Commission in France. Translated from Der Abolitionist. In "The Shield," October, 1909.
"Sentinel" Tracts. The Licensing of Sin in India.
Service de Sûreté publique et de Salubrité. Rapport. Brussels, 1880.
Stansfeld, Right Hon. James, M.P., The Failure of the Contagious Diseases Acts as Proved, etc., London.
Stansfeld, Right Hon. James, M.P., Lord Kimberley's Defence of the Government Brothel System, etc. 1882.
Stead, W. T., Josephine E. Butler: A Life Sketch. London, 1888.
Taylor, C. Bell, M.D., The Statistical Result of the Contagious Diseases Acts as Deduced from the Parliamentary Papers. 1872.
Turner, George Kibbe. The Daughters of the Poor. In McClure's Magazine, November, 1909.
White Slave Traffic. In Pall Mall Gazette, July, 1885.

Part III. The Prevention of Venereal Disease

CHAPTER I

UNDERLYING PRINCIPLES OF PREVENTION

PROSTITUTION TO BE PREVENTED. The genuine prevention of venereal disease is only made possible by the prevention of prostitution. Prostitution cannot be retained and the diseases fostered in it be eliminated. Prostitution must be rooted out, unless modern civilised states are content to look forward to the same fate which befell ancient Rome.

The English women, as they worked on through their crusade, came to see what at first they had not realised, that what they were making war upon was actually the social institution of prostitution itself. Thirty-five years ago Mrs. Butler said, in a public address: "That we are, and have been all along, contending for more than the mere repeal of these unjust and unholy Acts of Parliament, is proved by certain signs which are becoming more and more clear and frequent."

130   Hygiene and Morality

She went on: "We were perhaps ourselves unconscious—some of us are probably yet unconscious—how great is the undertaking upon which we have entered," and she then added with great solemnity, "it only very gradually dawned with perfect clearness on my mind that it is the old, the inveterate, the deeply-rooted evil of prostitution itself against which we are destined to make war." Mrs. Butler was saddened by seeing that some men, who had aided her against the special tyranny of special laws, grew cold and fell away as they found that her purpose struck at the very existence of prostitution itself. But her ideals of lofty personal and civic morality are now justified and sustained by those discoveries and teachings of science which, in her day, were still unheard, as to the causation and propagation of venereal diseases and even more so as to heredity. What men will not refrain from under persuasion alone, they will learn to refrain from under the warnings of medical and sanitary science, when these teachings are widely disseminated throughout all social circles. Just as the great mass of people have responded with readiness and intelligence to the doctrine of the preventability of tuberculosis, so, when they understand, will they respond to the doctrine of the far easier preventability of venereal diseases.

Even if the immoral projects of some writers could be realised in the use of immunising vaccines or serums to enable men to continue indulgence with greater security, venereal diseases would still continue to exist while prostitution exists, and, unless every man and woman in the world could be so vaccinated, there would be no security that the reckless, the unthinking, and the unsuspecting innocent would not continue to fall victims to, and to become carriers of, these deadly scourges. Nor is it credible that the aroused moral sense of humanity would consent to the general compulsory vaccination of syphilis and gonorrhœa as it does to that of smallpox, because moral sense, or even plain every-day common-sense, will distinguish between diseases which cannot be extirpated by moral living and the exertion of self-control through the power of the intelligent will, and diseases which can be so extirpated. The deliberate use of immunising substances with the intention of making it hygienically safe for men to continue a brutal misuse of women such as falls far below the practices of animals in vileness, could only be tolerated in a society that was ready for its own ruin. If such a practice is to be recommended as desirable for military recruits, and regarded as hopeful by military authorities, then this is only one more reason for the imperative social necessity of replacing the outworn military ideals by those of a higher conception of human brotherhood.[1]

However great may be the boon science has to bring to the present victims of immorality in the form of merciful antitoxins which may shear disease of its worst terrors, as diphtheria has been shorn by the serum of Behring, it will nevertheless remain true that real prevention does not rest there. Dr. Prince A. Morrow, president of the American Society of Sanitary and Moral Prophylaxis, says: "It is not a question of making prostitution safe, but of preventing the making of prostitutes." This lofty teaching is now being reiterated by ever larger numbers of the foremost leaders of medical science.

There are, in truth, no other diseases whose absolute prevention lies so wholly in human power as these.

---

[1] Various articles and books have been written on this line, which the author hesitates to mention because of the possibility of seeming to recommend them.

Principles of Prevention

KNOWLEDGE IS ESSENTIAL. The first essential in a campaign of prevention is full, open, and serious instruction for all classes of society upon the situation as it exists to-day; instruction without exaggeration, but also without concealment, of the present extent of disease of venereal origin, and with the most emphatic and positive information upon the real source of danger in prostitution. It will be found that not only is the extent to which venereal diseases have been allowed to prey upon the national stock utterly undreamed of by great numbers of highly intelligent persons, but that their very existence is, to thousands of others, only the vaguest hearsay, while to thousands more absolutely unknown. Now, as in combating typhoid fever and the plague the first thing needful is that all shall know that there are such diseases, whence their origin, and how they may be cut off at their source, so it is essential that every citizen shall know that there are venereal diseases, where they arise, and how they may be exterminated.

Therefore, a wide-spread campaign of popular education must be the first movement made. This has already been begun by the national societies founded for the purpose, and, as their task is a most difficult one, they should have the active support of every right thinking man and woman. Extreme difficulties meet this movement at the outset, arising from the peculiarly personal origin of these diseases, the prevailing false modesty as to the reproductive functions, and the generally dense ignorance of the physiology and hygiene of the generative organs. The vulgar prudery and hypocrisy of a past age compelled all such subjects to be tabooed, as being indelicate or improper. Perhaps this point of view has been encouraged by those whose interests were selfish or evil; certainly nothing could better serve such interests than the veil of silence and the cloak of embarrassment drawn over subjects so vital, pertaining to functions by nature so sacred, but by man so horribly debased. The function of reproduction, for which the organs of generation have been evolved, though it has been dragged through the mire of vulgar thoughts and cruel abuse, is yet the noblest, as it should be the most held in reverence of all human powers. Reproduction is natural, and should no more be regarded vulgarly than are the changes of the seasons. It is a type and symbol of immortality. It is indeed a present and visible immortality,

Principles of Prevention 135

and its humble physical phenomena should never obscure its exalted significance. The generative act should only be performed in the sincerity of aspiration to bring a new being into the world. Such being the truth, the depravity of exercising so miraculous a power for the sole desire of a passing pleasure of sensation, often combining with it drunkenness, and orgies in which all human dignity and decency are cast away, is so complete that the decay and fall of nations would seem to need no further explanation.

The generative organs do not suffer by non-use. This statement is now being emphasised with great earnestness by our foremost medical teachers. Nor does the general health suffer by their non-use. This is also emphasised, and is the basis of the modern scientific teaching upon sex hygiene that is now being given to young men in the universities of many countries.

It must be seen to that no children are allowed to grow up in the future in ignorance or with secret vulgarised notions of sex physiology. The simple truth, told them little by little from the earliest age at which they begin to ask questions and in a way which will appeal to their idealism; then later teaching in the schools in biology, physiology, and nature study, will go far toward prevention, by introducing a new ideal. The teaching of older boys and girls should point to their responsibilities to future generations.

As a woman physician has well said, young men who might be deaf to the appeal of an individualistic morality may be moved to response by the presentation of their debt to race and country.

The education of fathers and mothers must, in the future, include the principles of heredity, the toxic effect of unholy passions upon temperament and character, and the study of eugenics, the new science for the improvement of the race of man.

First and last, women need to be encouraged to revolt against a status of political and legal inferiority which is the direct cause of their economic and social degradation.

PRACTICAL MEANS OF PREVENTION. These may be divided into two classes: one, the means of individual care or personal prevention of disease as such; the other, the means of social or deep-lying prevention of the *causes* of disease. The former is the more immediate, the latter more fundamental. The former will soon prove to be insufficient without the intervention of the latter. A comparison with other forms of infectious disease may serve as illustration.

When typhoid fever is epidemic, all persons are warned to boil their drinking water; yet Boards of Health are not satisfied with that individual precaution, but hold it necessary to protect remote sources of water supply, no matter how great the initial outlay of money.

In the warfare against tuberculosis, the first thing taught is the proper disposal of sputum, but no one rests satisfied with that, and presently it becomes evident that the whole question of housing and of occupation presses for solution, bringing with it the details of rent, of land monopoly, and of private ownership of the means of industry. Or, just as, in the expectation of raising a certain kind of crop, the farmer begins several years in advance by planting something quite different, or by expending capital on accessories, so must the social prevention of the social evil with its train of disease be arrived at by remote and indirect routes.

The personal precautions, being the most immediate, may be considered first.

PERSONAL PREVENTION OF VENEREAL DISEASE: CHILDHOOD. From earliest childhood there must be prevention of all habits known as self-abuse or masturbation, namely, all stimulation of the delicate nerve centres and fibres that are connected with the genital organs. Every nurse knows that such habits may arise even with babies, in complete innocence, of course, and that, if not checked, they may be less innocently continued by older children with grave danger both to health and morals. Mothers should be impressed with the dangers of this habit to the delicate and undeveloped nervous system of the child. Many do not know how real these dangers are, and regard the habit as an unimportant one, believing that it will be outgrown, as sometimes it may be. Nurses should teach the routine of absolute cleanliness of the parts, the avoidance of overwarm clothing, of idle luxurious living, of rich stimulating food, and above all, of alcoholic drinks for children, as all of these tend to excite the nervous system, while local irritants, such as uncleanliness or thick clumsy clothing, may act directly upon the nerves of the skin. Children should sleep in beds alone, with plenty of fresh air, and, if necessary to break up a tendency to self-handling, their hands should be so confined as to prevent tendency from becoming habit. Mothers should provide regular, skilled medical inspection for all children, that no abnormal condition may be overlooked. Sometimes such cases require surgical interference. The hygiene of the older child calls for ample physical and manual training, daily bathing with cool water, friction, and rough towels; regularity of all excretory functions; fresh air and not too much sedentary or solitary or monotonous occupation. In talking with mothers upon these subjects, nurses should have fortified themselves by careful instructions from the wisest medical men or women. Sensational prophecy of the possible results of masturbation may do great harm, yet negligence or timidity in controlling it may do even more. It is important that all mothers should understand that the younger the child is who forms the habit the more injurious is the practice in its effects upon the nervous system. Furthermore, it is the conviction of Dr. Morrow that masturbation tends to incline its victims toward immoral habits and leads young men to debauchery.

Dr. Blackwell, in her book, *The Human Element in Sex*, deals instructively with masturbation, specifying its chief evils as, 1, the injury to the mind through the nervous system, and, 2, the danger of habit-formation with resultant loss of self-control, with all the dangers that follow upon this loss of mastery over one's self, even to the destruction of health, insanity, or suicide. She says in another place: "Precocious physical development hinders moral development."

Löwenfeld, in discussing mental working power, says that it is oftener injured by masturbation than by excesses, adding:

and it is not always a case of very early or excessive masturbation; in many cases of this habit there are also painful reflections, such as self-reproach, self-accusation, anxiety for consequences, recollection of religious teachings, which affect the nervous system and through it the mental working power.

OLDER CHILDREN. For older children there should be definite warnings of the dangers which they may meet, as carefully and explicitly given as directions in taking a perilous journey. To leave little girls, especially, in ignorance of what these dangers are, is as wicked as it would be to expose them to wild beasts. Such warnings should be given at an early age. The little girl of twelve has a simple seriousness and sagacity,

Principles of Prevention

which may be looked for in vain if she remains untaught and undisciplined up to sixteen or seventeen, when youthful gaiety often runs into recklessness.

Such warnings need not cloud the happiness of childhood more than other necessary knowledge of danger which is likely to be met, and even if it does, better that than the tragic fate which now overtakes thousands of little girls. That kind of sentimentality which regards the ignorance of children in the face of the worst of perils as desirable and lovely, is a sickly and unsafe, it may be even a treacherous sentimentality. It would at least seem to be beyond contradiction that the age at which the laws cease giving protection to little girls should be the age at which they are to be armed with the knowledge which will help them to protect themselves.

YOUTH. Equally criminal is it to let the boys go to boarding-school or college without the most serious and intimate counsel and warnings against the horrible diseases lurking amidst the "wild oats" that they may thoughtlessly sow.

It is estimated by the records of the sickness insurance system of Germany that 25% of university students become infected with venereal diseases. We have no such statistics to guide us, but the writer has learned from the personal knowledge of the head of a large hospital in a great university centre, of the numbers of young men who come in for treatment for loathsome diseases. A painful feature of this calamity is that "the mothers are never told the truth; the fathers come and some reassuring falsehood is sent home." It is thus evident that, in such cases, the mere fact of the mother knowing the truth is greatly dreaded. Therefore, if it could be certain that all mothers would learn the truth, is it not likely that a powerful deterrent to evil courses in university life might be brought into play? If this is the result of silence and ignorance, the questions arise: "Is this really shielding the sanctity of home life? Are not these mothers guilty of a serious shirking of duty by not knowing, if their knowing would mean even partial prevention?"

EARLY ADULT LIFE. It is a hopeful sign that the ancient heresy of "physical necessity" for irregular indulgence by men, so long upheld by them, tacitly assented to by women, and even sometimes taught by high medical authorities, is now being gradually repudiated and denied by the most eminent physicians and hygienists. To maintain it has been, indeed, an insult to all those men whose lives are and have been pure, and one must wonder that such men have so long permitted so detestable a doctrine to go unchallenged. Young men may now be taught, with all the authority of science, that the same virtue which is desirable for their sisters is good for them, and that "physical necessity," like drug habits, only grows coarser and ranker by indulgence and weakening of the will power. Self-control is an evidence of a strong and manly nature and of a well-balanced physical endowment.

MARRIAGE. Medical statistics show that the vast majority of all innocently contracted cases of venereal disease are those contracted by wives and children through the institution of marriage: that fifty per cent. of the sterility of wives and from twenty to twenty-five per cent. of the sterility of husbands is caused by the *gonococcus:* that a large per cent. of miscarriages and a heavy infant mortality are due to the *Spirochæte pallida:* that fully eighty per cent. of blindness from birth and twenty-five per cent. of all blindness is gonorrhœal: that the secondary symptoms of inherited syphilis often cause loss of sight or hearing: that from fifty to seventy-five per cent. of all gynecological operations, often involving amputation of the female organs of generation, and an indefinite proportion of all cases of chronic, life-long invalidism in women result from the deadly power of persistence of the *gonococcus* and its tendency to remain latent in the male organs, suddenly to kindle an acute inflammation in the virgin tissues to which it may gain access: it is therefore plain that the most extreme precautions of personal prevention need to be taken before the risk of marriage is run. No parent should allow a daughter to marry without securing authentic proof that the promised husband is free from disease. This is incontestably a duty of parents of the utmost gravity and importance, neglecting which all their previous care, expense, and nurture lavished on the daughter may go for naught. An honourable and virtuous man will willingly give such testimony, and might rightly demand on his side assurances from the parents as to their daughter's inheritance. Such inquiries are not impossible. They could all be conducted by

Principles of Prevention 145

the trusted physicians of one or both families with entire privacy and dignity. Fathers find ways to inform themselves of the business standing of prospective sons-in-law, and health is far more precious than money.

What personal prevention can there be for an innocent partner in marriage, if in later years infection is brought to her from prostitution? It would seem that here, as in the case of the college boy, the knowledge that the truth would surely become known might in many cases act as a deterrent. At present the victim (usually the wife) is kept in ignorance of the real cause of her illness. Certainly, if there is any inalienable right of the individual, it is to know what is the matter with one when one is ill. But at present two barriers are interposed: one is the general ignorance of the laity in matters of health preservation; the other is medical reticence. Only when women have sufficient general knowledge of health and disease, and courage to insist on the truth and to accept it when offered, can the second barrier be broken down. Already many physicians are chafing against the shackles of the "medical secret," and they are sometimes severely blamed for their share in the general blindfolding of the public in regard to venereal diseases. Yet to speak the truth in individual cases exposes them to suits-at-law and other most trying experiences. It can, however, hardly be doubted that the certainty of truth being known would in time have a salutary preventive effect upon married men. It would at least be a simple justice to their victims.

PREVENTION OF ACCIDENTAL INFECTION. Remembering the characteristics of the *Spirochæte pallida*, its extreme virulence while living, but short life period outside the body; and those of the *gonococcus*, with its equal or even greater virulence and perhaps somewhat greater tenacity of life outside the body; remembering that neither is conveyed by dust or through the air, but only by material objects, it should be possible for every one to guard against accidental infection, without suffering from exaggerated alarm. Common drinking cups, as in railway cars and public places, should be absolutely avoided. Individuals should carry their own cups. Progressive railroads are now providing individual drinking cups of paper, to be used once and then thrown away. They should be demanded of every public service cor-

Principles of Prevention 147

poration. Towels, too, in common use, must always be regarded as possible carriers. They should never be applied to the face and eyes unless freshly laundered. In general, it should be a matter of universal practice never to rub or even touch the eyes except with a clean piece of linen—never with the fingers or finger nails, as they carry all manner of infectious germs.

The face should not be washed directly from basins that are used indiscriminately, especially for rinsing the mouth. Rubbing the face with a clean wet towel may be substituted in travelling.

Eating utensils which have been washed and dried may be regarded as probably safe, yet in many places it would no doubt be an added security to carry one's own fork and spoon. The fresh cleanliness of bed linen cannot be too carefully looked into when travelling. The conditions of public laundries should also be a matter of investigation by housekeepers. The seats of public water-closets may always be regarded as being more or less doubtful, and when used, may be covered with a clean piece of paper. Many cases of gonorrhœa are caused by the dirty or ill-kept seats of public conveniences, especially in crowded places. Public bath tubs should be used with precautions of thorough cleansing, and if doubtful, had better be let alone. No object should ever be put to the lips or eyes which may have been so handled by other persons, such as pencils, pens, sticks, etc. To put money into the mouth should be forbidden by the Boards of Health. The importance of having individual towels, face-cloths, napkins, utensils, etc., is now generally recognised in institutions, homes, asylums, and schools. Such articles are, if used in common, of course capable of conveying many kinds of infection, and it will be seen that the avoidance of mechanical contagion of venereal disease is much like that of tuberculosis and pus diseases, the chief difference being that of the absence of danger from dust in the one and its great danger in the others.

In caring for cases of venereal diseases, nurses and others should observe as rigid a technic of disinfection as in diphtheria or other acute infectious fevers. All discharges from the mucous membranes, ulcerated or suppurating tissues, eyes, mouth, or nose should be received on clean waste material and promptly burned. Clothing and bed linen should be boiled or sterilised, then well sunned and aired. The danger of infecting

Principles of Prevention 149

laundresses by unsterilised clothing should always be remembered. Complete isolation of dishes and utensils should be observed and they should be periodically boiled. Patients with mucous patches should never expectorate carelessly, for, though the dried germs are not dangerous, there is always the possibility of direct contact in some manner before the death of the germs. Nor should such patients sneeze or cough without carefully protecting their surroundings by covering the nose or mouth. This, indeed, should be the usual routine for all persons at all times.

It is the right of every nurse, for self-protection, to know what she is taking care of, and it should be impressed upon all nurses that they must invariably insist upon knowing the diagnosis in the cases they care for. It has not infrequently happened that nurses, kept by the attending physician in ignorance of the venereal origin of patients' maladies, have contracted them. It is also true that if all nurses were sufficiently well taught and trained, it should be second nature with them to avoid all infectious contact. The proper precautions being observed, nurses and all others should comprehend clearly that there is no danger whatever from the simple presence of cases of venereal disease amidst other people, and no more danger in caring for them than there is with cases of ordinary sepsis. Accidental infection arises solely from ignorance; this cannot be too strongly emphasised. Proof is amply given by the results of well-managed venereal wards, where infection of attendants and nurses does not occur. French experts have recently recommended the inclusion of adult venereal patients (with the possible exception of extreme cases) in the general wards of hospitals for the sake of the better moral and mental influence, and explain that the recommendation is perfectly practicable because with the proper technic of care such patients need not be regarded as dangerous from the stand-point of infection.

In conclusion it should be remembered that there are probably no other diseases where early and competent medical advice is more all-important. If quackery is always a blunder, here it is a fatal one, and nurses should use their whole power as teachers to impress this on their communities. All the social circumstances connected with the time of cure and return of such patients to normal life make the necessity for the best medical oversight one of paramount importance.

SOCIAL PREVENTION OF PROSTITUTION. In order to approach social methods of preventing prostitution in a perfectly intelligent way there should first be three main lines of inquiry, which can here be simply indicated, in the briefest fashion, as lines on which there is work waiting for women to do. They are:

First, to discover the extent of prostitution. Second, to ascertain its various reasons for existence,—what they are and how much diversity they have to show. Third, to penetrate to the social arrangements in which these reasons are imbedded, and to see how much there is here that is artificial and needless.

The right attitude of mind with which to undertake such inquiry is, that it is rational to believe that prostitution and its resultant diseases can be reduced to a minimum, and that it is possible for that minimum to be discovered. To be convinced that it can be and inflexibly determined that it must be discovered is no more visionary or theoretical than it has been in the past to believe in all the dawning possibilities of human progress. There was a time when it was thought that the plague, typhus, smallpox, and other infectious diseases could not be conquered.

Science has indeed not banished any of these ills entirely from the earth, but it has given society the knowledge of how to keep them down to their lowest terms.

THE EXTENT OF PROSTITUTION. It is doubtful whether correct figures could be obtained at present of the entire extent of prostitution. This would be the first task to undertake in initiating an aggressive campaign against the institution as such. But, taking the world over, being guided by the statements that are made by officials and social students regarding single cities and countries, it is hardly doubtful that there are, in all, several million women set aside in this life. It was stated at the Brussels congress, conservatively, that there were fifty thousand in England. Taber Johnson estimates the number in the United States at about half a million who are in houses of ill-fame, and believes there may be as many more outside of such places. In exerting the imagination to picture this number of women pariahs and to call them together in one mass before the mental vision in order to personify them, and to consider the problem of their relation to disease, it is to be remembered that this dreary race does not perpetuate itself. Prostitutes quickly become sterile, and few leave children. Their lives, moreover, are very short. Some authorities estimate the average life of the prostitute as ten years; some believe it to be even less,—a five-year average. Between these two estimates it may be possible there is a mean, but even this is sufficiently short, especially as it does not signify their working life, so to speak, but the actual span of life. In from five to ten years they die, many from pneumonia, tuberculosis, alcoholism, and suicide, while practically all of them, says Dr. Morrow, finally become cases of venereal disease of one form or another. Now, if it were only this half-million or so of women in our own country who were doomed to early disease and premature death for no better or more useful reason than to gratify the brutal and selfish lusts of men that will finally destroy those very men themselves, this alone would be a disgrace to modern hygiene and civilisation. It may be illustrated by supposing that a half-million women were set apart at any one time in our great country to be infected with leprosy or to be compelled to die of diphtheria. All the health boards of the country would be in a state of desperate activity, and the daily press would find no headlines sufficiently sensational. But it is actually even worse than this, for, in order to fill the vacancies caused by disease and death, some 50,000 fresh and once at least pure, clean, and innocent young girls must be annually drafted into this death-dealing business.

Solely as a matter of public health, without regarding moral considerations for a moment, this is a danger of paramount importance, yet it meets with less concern from health boards than half-a-dozen smallpox cases. Indeed, the discovery of one smallpox case is telegraphed all over the country, but the fact that numbers of young girls are set aside yearly to die of venereal disorders and their tragic accompaniments is ignored by sanitary departments and the press.

From this point of view, too, the extent of prostitution as the source of venereal disease must be noted in the light of the computation of experts, that for every abandoned woman there are at the least five profligate men. Dr. Morrow estimates, from carefully collected data, that, of the young men in this country reaching their sixteenth year (numbering 770,000 annually), at least sixty per cent. or over 450,000 of each

Principles of Prevention

year's cohort, will, at some time of life, become infected with venereal disease, and that twenty per cent. of such infection will occur before the end of the twenty-first year.

REASONS FOR THE EXISTENCE OF PROSTITUTION. What are these reasons and how diverse are they? The statements of the United States District-Attorney, as well as of speakers at the Brussels conferences, indicating that about four fifths of all prostitutes are unwillingly such, though painful, have a hopeful aspect, as they point definitely to the conclusion that prostitution is capable of being reduced to an easily controllable minimum. If these four fifths of unwilling members of the sad army could be withheld from entering this life, it would not be an insoluble problem to deal with the remaining fifth. Distributed, as they would be, over the whole country, the number of "chronic or persevering" prostitutes with which each community had to deal would not be an unmanageable number. If they were irreclaimable, they could be kept in colonies, tenderly and wisely cared for, as are the insane and feeble-minded. If this ideal method should be too advanced, then, when there were really only the

Hygiene and Morality

prostitutes by preference to consider, and then only, might direct legislation of a punitive character for women be spoken of without bitter injustice and wrong.

The only true prevention for such chronic or determined evil-doers, and the prevention that the future must show how to apply, is, not to have them born. Who can say, now, that they are not the inevitable hereditary consequences of their parents' sexual excesses?

Unwilling victims of a stupid social order should not be regarded as true prostitutes, but as sacrifices, as human loss and waste due to pure mismanagement. The underlying reason for their lapse is poverty or the unequal struggle against want. All medical and social experts who have studied this problem agree that prostitution is a disease of poverty. Testimony on this point is so abundant that it is not necessary to prove the point here, but it may be recalled that the favourite buttress for the arguments of those who uphold prostitution and licensed vice is the dictum that "there must always be prostitution because there will always be poverty."

Poverty, then, must be so far eradicated or at least so far mitigated that it cannot honestly be

Principles of Prevention

given as an explanation of prostitution. This is the social prevention of venereal diseases which are fostered in prostitution.

It will now be clear how far-reaching and remote are the paths along which the prevention of venereal diseases must be pursued. They lead even farther than the road to the prevention of typhoid fever, which follows the water-courses back to the pure springs of the head-waters. And they are obstructed by the same obstacles in the mercenary interests that have become parasitic; but besides all these they are blocked by one obstacle which no other contagious disease has ever had to meet, namely, the selfish and hitherto uncontrolled pleasure of indulgence of the individual man. The prevalence and power of this pleasure-lust make it hopeless to expect that a majority of men will give it up themselves of their own volition; and vain, therefore, is it to look to their management for prevention of prostitution. It will be found again, as Mrs. Butler found, that many will readily lop off the worst manifestations of this institution, such as the white slave traffic, who will never whole-heartedly undertake the eradication of the institution itself. Already this is clear in the articles which are now appearing in the periodicals and daily papers upon the white slave trade; horror of the trade is freely expressed, with shame and contrition for its existence, but one may search vainly through the lay press for any bugle-call to men to put an end to prostitution. This must be the work of women, and to do it they must possess the instrument which is as indispensable in controlling the acts of legislatures, which lie behind all social conditions, as is the microscope to the physician in his research work, or the scissors to the mother who is cutting out her children's clothes.

ENFRANCHISEMENT OF WOMEN THE FIRST STEP. Long ago Dr. Taylor said that every method had been tried for the prevention of venereal disease except one, and that was the teaching of continence to young men. But Dr. Taylor was wrong, though a good and noble man; for in his day no one had ever dreamed of trying the remedy of giving power and authority to the mothers of young men. And it is passing strange that so few even of the men sincerely desirous of wiping these scourges of disease from the earth should think of this remedy, even when, as at the Brussels conferences, they have racked their brains for suggestions and have put forth some that seem almost childish in their grasping at straws. For now it is possible to see the beginnings of what women will do with this matter of prostitution and venereal disease when they have full political power. To-day, the only parts of the world where this combined problem is progressing toward solution are those parts where women have been in possession of the ballot long enough to show some results of their direct influence.[1]

Only the determination of women who are politically free, expressed through the machinery of government by the right use of popular government's only instrument, the ballot, can effect the downfall of prostitution as a social and commercial institution. Some broad-minded men there are who do see this. Professor James Stuart said to Dr. Emily Ford, of England, when she asked what could be done to stop commercialised vice, *"Go on trying for woman suffrage"*; while in our own country there are medical members of the American Society of Sanitary and Moral Prophylaxis who take the same position.

SOCIAL STEPS IN PREVENTION. There must be

[1] See Appendix B.

full and ample protection for children from the very cradle,—yes, even earlier. It must be possible for every child to be well born, and the pregnant mother must be protected first from want, poverty, and sweated labour.

Child labour must be abolished and child-culture substituted for it. Children that are forced into the labour market are almost foredoomed to prostitution and venereal disease because their enfeeblement and premature exhaustion weakens will power, retards useful education, and warps their natures, whilst the exposure to all sorts of moral dangers cannot be avoided by little wage-slaves. The need of ample legal protection for little girls has been sufficiently shown by the facts of the "age of consent" laws. These laws and the resistance of legislatures to their amendment, show only too plainly that they have been intentionally framed and kept, not for the protection of girls, but for the protection of men while keeping an open door through which a sufficient supply of young girls may be continually passed into ruin. This is a painful reflection, but it is the only possible conclusion from the facts.

But further, for the real protection of girls not only legislation, but vigilant administration and unswerving enforcement of law must be had. Now, the former, or some appearance of it, may indeed be secured as a concession from men, but the latter can never be hoped for until women possess the same public and legal powers that men now possess.[1] This is a point that is almost invariably overlooked. The flippant query so often heard, "Shall we have women police?" needs to be answered seriously in the affirmative; women are urgently, desperately needed as police wherever young children and growing creatures are out in the world, and the time may not be far off when such police, with the training of the nurse or the teacher, shall be more numerous than those we are now familiar with. Then, and for the first time, there will be real "morals police." Widowed mothers must not be compelled to act as father and mother both, by being driven to earn their children's bread outside the home while trying to keep their little ones in the home. Through this double burden women have been driven to the streets, or their little ones have found the way there. There are seas of sentimentality poured forth about the home,—but it never seems to be the home of the working people

[1] See Appendix C.

that is meant. Yet these are the majority of the homes. To one of America's deepest-hearted and most clear-seeing women, a sight that seemed too intolerable to be borne was the sight of a working mother whose abundant milk dripped to the floor as she scrubbed business offices for sixteen hours a day. Who can tell how such sins against family life will end?

The real protection of mothers and of children will be, as to prostitution and venereal disease, what the protection of the head-waters is to typhoid fever; for, as Judge Lindsay's recent true story has shown, *it is absolutely essential for the children to be ruined at a tender age, if a vicious and corrupt class is to be maintained.*[1]

The fundamental and crying need in the protection of older girls is a living wage. It is only too well known that employers in every country where women are disfranchised have not infrequently given to their young employees, along with their wage pittances, the suggestion that it is always open to them to earn more without difficulty. The researches recently made by the National Consumers' League into the relation between the cost of living and the wages paid

[1] See Appendix D.

Principles of Prevention 163

to girls in industry in New York City, striking as they have been in their demonstration of gross inequality, give cause for added thought in view of the official information that that city is the centre of the white slave trade.[1]

Hours of work need to be shortened for all workers. Overwork, monotony, and chronic fatigue make all work hateful and destroy healthful ideals, while the long hours of work leave no time for natural enjoyment or pleasure in life.

It is often said, as a piece of superior wisdom, that men cannot be made moral by law. It is only superficially true. Conditions which make young boys and girls, young women and men, or older women and men immoral by necessity can be and should be altered by the law. Indeed they must be, because the whole modern social structure rests finally on the support given to it by laws. Intelligent social legislation, when rightly enforced, is like the fence that keeps marauders out of an orchard. Vainly does the gardener put forth his best work if the fence is not there and the despoilers are. If we could get rid of marauders, we might do without fences, as the French gardens need none.

[1] See Appendix E.

The influence of unenfranchised woman is nullified and frustrated precisely as are the efforts of the unprotected gardener. Her fence will be the ballot, but she must build it herself. The marauders who threaten her are all the vicious and dangerous elements among men who know that her supremacy means the ultimate disappearance of that social evil on which they base all their profitable exploitation of the young and the helpless. These enemies, though the most venomous, are the most silent; they are never heard in arguments against woman suffrage.[1]

English women writers, medical women and the leaders of the suffrage movement both in England and in our own country, declare in the most explicit terms that the real hostility to the advance of women comes from those who exploit prostitution, while, on the other hand, at the foundation of the terrible earnestness of the women of England to gain the Parliamentary franchise is the burning and unflinching determination to free womanhood from this disgrace. In this country the story is the same, though not so well understood by the great mass of women.

The fear of the "bad woman's vote" has long

[1] See Appendix F.

been dangled as a spectre before the eyes of timid good women. How fictitious this fear is may be realised by summing up the testimony proving that eighty per cent. of the "bad women" need not have been bad; that almost all prostitution is commercial, and that its promoters rely chiefly for their supplies on the ruin of children of tender years, eking out with young girls snared in their silly and thoughtless age; that the white slave trade is now and always has been supported and protected by men politically corrupt; that in Colorado, where all women vote, the "bad women" actually cast just one third of one per cent. of the vote of Denver[1]; that the women of that State, though in the minority, have succeeded in placing model statutes for the protection and training of children upon the books, and have helped to maintain in power against bitter enemies the one man fearless enough to enforce and reinforce them, while in the three other enfranchised states not a word is ever heard about a "bad" vote; that in New Zealand prostitution has been reduced to its lowest terms, while commercialised vice is practically extinct there. Well did Dr.

[1] Dr. Aylesworth, in his Carnegie Hall address, Nov. 17, 1909.

Aylesworth say, "These women [the prostitutes] exert a hundred fold more influence upon politicians through their business than through their ballots."

A NEW IDEAL NEEDED. A new ideal needs to be formed; an ideal of the worth and dignity of human life, and of a commanding place and power that must be assumed by women in all that pertains to the cherishing and ennobling of the race. This ideal must be built upon the single standard of sex morality and it must be attained by a gradual process of assumption of knowledge and authority by women, to the end that they may finally produce a nobler and a finer race of men.

SOURCES OF MATERIAL USED IN THE PREPARATION OF PART III.

Abbott, Edith, Women in Industry. 1909.
American Society of Sanitary and Moral Prophylaxis. Publications. 9 East 42d St., New York City.
    The Boy Problem: For Parents and Teachers.
    The Young Man's Problems: For Teachers.
    The Relations of Social Diseases with Marriage, and their Prophylaxis.
    How My Uncle, the Doctor, Instructed Me in Matters of Sex.
    Health and the Hygiene of Sex: for College Students.
Anthony, Susan B., and Harper, Ida Husted, History of Woman Suffrage. 4 vols.
Arendt, Sister Henriette (for five years assistant police officer in Stuttgart, in charge of women prisoners before and after their discharge), Menschen die den Pfad Verloren. Stuttgart, 1907.
Aves, Ernest, Report to the Secretary of State for the Home Department on the Wages Boards and Industrial Conciliation and Arbitration Acts of Australia and New Zealand. London, 1908. (Blue Book.)
Blackwell, Elizabeth, M.D., Counsel to Parents on the Moral Education of Their Children. 1880.
Blackwell, Elizabeth, M.D., The Human Element in Sex, 1884.
Blackwell, Elizabeth, M.D., The Laws of Life, with Special Reference to the Physical Education of Girls. 1852.
Blackwell, Elizabeth, M.D., Medicine and Morality.
Blackwell, Elizabeth, M.D., Pioneer Work in Opening the Medical Profession to Women. 1896.

Hygiene and Morality

Blackwell, Elizabeth, M.D., The Religion of Health.
Blackwell, Elizabeth, M.D., Wrong and Right Methods of Dealing with Social Evil. (No date; about 1860–70.)
Broadhead, State Regulation of Labour and Labour Disputes in New Zealand. 1908.
Bureau of Labour, Labour Conditions in Australia (Bulletin, Vol. X., 1905).
Bureau of Labour, Minimum Wages Act of 1908 in New South Wales, p. 86. (Bulletin No. 80. January, 1909.)
Conference on the Care of Dependent Children, Washington, D. C., January 25, 26, 1909. Proceedings.
Eugenics Education Society. Publications. London.
Immigration Committee, Report. Importing Women for Immoral Purposes. (Senate Document No. 196.)
Jacobi, Mary Putnam, M.D., Common-Sense Applied to Woman Suffrage. New York, 1894.
Kelley, Florence, Some Ethical Gains Through Legislation. New York, 1905.
Löwenfeld, Die geistige Arbeitskraft. In Grenzfragen des Nerven und Seelenlebens. Vol. vi.
Macrosty, State Arbitration and the Minimum Wage in Australasia. In Trade Unionism and Labour Problems, edited with an Introduction by John R. Commons, p. 195. New York, 1905.
Martindale, L., M.D., Under the Surface. Brighton, England.
National American Woman Suffrage Association. Political Equality Leaflets:
    Blackwell, Alice Stone, Fruits of Equal Suffrage, i., ii.
    Holder, Lady, Equal Suffrage in Australia.
    Kelley, Florence, Woman Suffrage: Its Relation to Working Women and Children.
    Macnaghten, R. E., Women's Vote in Australia.
    Nathan, Maud, Wage Earner and the Ballot.
    Russell, Charles Edward, Woman Suffrage in New Zealand.
    Wells, Mrs. Borrman, New Zealand's Experience. '
New York Probation Association. First Report. 165 W. 10th St., New York City.

Sources of Material Used

Oregon and Illinois Briefs relating to Overwork. The Consumers' League, 105 E. 22d St., New York City.

Roosevelt's (President) Homes Commission Report. (Senate Document No. 644.)

Royal Commission on the Poor Laws. Minority Report. London, 1909.

University of London, Eugenics Laboratory Lecture Series. London.

APPENDIX A

ATTEMPTS TO INTRODUCE REGULATION INTO THE UNITED STATES

ST. LOUIS: Attempt made in 1870 under pretext of suppressing prostitution. The words "or regulate" introduced into a clause of the city charter established a system of supervised vice which continued until 1874, when it was abolished by the force of public indignation.

CALIFORNIA: In 1871 the legislature had a bill brought before it for legalising and regulating vice. The wife of a member drew up and had presented a bill identical with the first except that the word "man" was substituted throughout where the word "woman" appeared in the original bill. The obnoxious bill was withdrawn.

CINCINNATI: In 1874 an attempt was made to regulate vice by enactment but it was defeated.

PENNSYLVANIA: In 1874 a bill was presented in the legislature for the State regulation of vice. Fifty-two medical men sent a noble protest, affirming the single moral standard. The bill was defeated.

DISTRICT OF COLUMBIA: Regulation by the Board of Health was proposed in 1875 and was defeated.

NEW YORK STATE: About the same date similar legislation brought before the legislature was defeated by the power of Elizabeth Cady Stanton, Susan B. Anthony, and their allies.

[Data taken from *A Comparative Survey of Laws*, etc., by Sheldon Ames.]

APPENDIX B

EXAMPLES OF THE KIND OF LEGISLATION WOMEN ARE ESPECIALLY INTERESTED IN AND WORK FOR

WYOMING: Equal pay to men and women teachers of equal qualification.

Age of protection for girls raised to 18.

Penalties for neglect, abuse, or cruelty shown to children.

Prohibition of the labour of boys under 14 in mines.

No cigarettes, liquor, or tobacco to be sold or given to persons under 16.

Free public kindergartens established.

Licensed gambling forbidden.

Provision for the care and custody of deserted or orphan children and children of infirm, indigent, or incompetent persons.

COLORADO: State home for dependent children established. Two of the five members of the board of managers must be women.

Provision that at least three out of six members of the board of county visitors shall be women.

Hygiene and Morality

Mothers made joint guardians of their children with the fathers [this equality of parents exists in only thirteen of the States of the Union].

Age of protection for girls raised to 18.

State industrial home for girls established; three of the five members of the board of managers to be women.

Protective care for the feeble-minded provided.

Woman physician placed on the board of the asylums for the insane.

Juvenile courts and truant schools established; education compulsory to the 16th year.

Union high schools established.

Advanced regulations for child labour and an eight-hour day for children of 16 or under.

Prohibition for over eight hours a day for women working in occupations that require standing.

To contribute to the delinquency of a child made a criminal offence.

IDAHO: Gambling made illegal.
Age of protection for girls raised to 18.
Industrial reform school established.
Equalisation of married women's rights in property.

UTAH: Equal pay for men and women teachers equally qualified.

Age of protection for girls raised to 18.

Sale or gift of cigarettes, tobacco, opium, or any other narcotic to persons under 18 forbidden.

Provisions for protection of children against neglect or ill treatment.

Free kindergartens established.

[The above examples have been taken from pamphlets by Alice Stone Blackwell: *Fruits of Equal Suffrage*, I. and II. Only those that are specially pertinent to the subject under discussion in the text have been chosen, whilst the pamphlets themselves give numerous other examples without assuming to show a complete list. It is pointed out that laws of this character are much better enforced where women are enfranchised. The leaflets are published by the National American Woman Suffrage Association, 505 Fifth Avenue, New York City.]

NEW ZEALAND: Legal standard of morality and conditions of divorce made the same for men and women.

Legal separation from worthless husbands obtainable summarily and without expense.

Testator's Family Maintenance Act prevents a man from willing away his property without making suitable provision for wife and family.

Old-age pensions for aged persons of both sexes; an old couple may receive a joint pension in their own home.

Government asylums for inebriates established.

Health of women workers and of workers of both sexes under 18 carefully protected; hours of labour and legal holidays with payment regulated [the eight-hour day is legal]; payment of wages to learners in trades secured and workers' compensation for accidents defined with great advantage to the working people.

Purer code of morals established by alterations in the criminal code.

Adoption of children regulated by law and baby farming prevented.

Industrial schools and technical schools established.

[From *Woman Suffrage in New Zealand*, published by the International Woman Suffrage Alliance. Leaflet No. 1.]

AUSTRALIA: On the federal domain the chief gains so far are:

Equal pay for equal work in government departments.

Naturalisation laws made equal for men and women.

Unified marriage and divorce bills.

Appendices

In the separate (Australian) states the gains are: wages boards; children's courts; old-age pensions; protection for wage-earning children; married women's property acts; aid for the illegitimate mother; reforms in the drink trade.

[From *Where Women have the Vote*, published by the National Union of Women's Suffrage Societies, 25 Victoria St., Westminster, London; quoting Miss Alice Zimmern's *Women's Suffrage in Many Lands*.]

APPENDIX C

SOME STATISTICS OF CRIMINAL ASSAULT UPON YOUNG GIRLS [1]

By Mary Burr, Delegate to the International Congress of Nurses of the National Council of Trained Nurses of Great Britain and Ireland.

Statistics are usually considered very dry, but when those figures mean ruined lives, as they do in this paper, then they assume an aspect which should command our very closest attention. In endeavouring to gather these statistics, it was originally intended to draw as far as possible upon private sources. These, however, proved inadequate, and a dozen different societies which deal with wronged women and children were approached for whatever information they could give.

The results proved somewhat curious; from only

[1] Read at the International Congress of Nurses, London, July, 1909. Reprinted in the *British Journal of Nursing*, Nov. 6, 1909.

two did I receive any definite information—the National Society for the Prevention of Cruelty to Children and the Church Penitentiary Association.

Of the other societies, six referred me to some one else, and even the National Vigilance Society, from which I expected much, referred me to the Director of Public Prosecutions; the remainder said they did not deal with such cases.

One lady flatly refused to furnish information which she considered private to a congress of which she knew nothing.

It made one wonder if this work, which so closely affects the national well-being, is a private preserve, reserved to those who work in it. It almost appears so. Information was sought on four points only:

1. The number of cases of criminal assault committed upon young girls and children.

2. The number of cases in which prosecution followed.

3. The result of the prosecution.

4. The ages of the victims.

The idea was to find out as far as possible the extent of this awful evil; what proportion of the offenders were punished and the degree of punishment inflicted, because, of various cases which had come to my knowledge, only a very small proportion were brought to justice. As so little information

180   Hygiene and Morality

was obtained from the societies from which I had hoped to gain so much, I took the advice of one secretary, and bought the Blue Book of Criminal Statistics, and here is the result.

Comparative statistics are given for 15 years from 1893 to 1907; the details of 1907 only are given. In those 15 years there were 2302 cases of defilement of girls under 13 years of age, and 2442 cases of defilement of girls under 16 years of age, making the terrible total of 4744 cases reported to the police.

Of these 3425 were tried—1660 for assault on girls under 13, the remaining 1765 being for girls under 16.

The details of the cases for 1907, which are included in the above figures, are as follows:—Reported to the police, 149 cases concerning girls under 13, and 178 concerning girls under 16; total, 327. Of these, 97 of the first and 135 of the latter were tried, a total of 232 cases, roughly about two thirds. Five cases were thrown out, 82 were acquitted, 145 convicted. The punishment of those convicted was penal servitude in 23 cases for terms varying from four to twenty years, five and seven years being the usual sentence; one man was flogged; the remainder received terms of imprisonment from fourteen days to two years.

One curious fact in this grim document is the distinction drawn between girls under and over 13.

All the sentences of penal servitude were given in the former cases, and not one in the latter; apparently a girl over 13 and under 16 may be treated in the most dastardly manner and the sentence be anything between fourteen days and two years.

This does not conclude the terrible sum of immorality among the males of this Christian land, for during the years quoted—1893 to 1907—there were also 3407 cases of rape, and 12,280 cases of indecent assault upon women over 16, reported to the police, altogether making the ghastly total of 15,687 cases reported, and with the 4744 cases under 16, we have the tremendous number of 20,431—an annual average for the fifteen years of 1362 women's lives wrecked. Such is the information from the Blue Book.

The Rev. Thomas George Cree, Hon. Secretary of the Church Penitentiary Association, sent me a very interesting little pamphlet, *Juvenile Immorality*, in which he states that he sent out a circular to all the homes and refuges on their list asking for the number of such children under 16 dealt with during the last three years (up to October, 1908). Replies from 40 penitentiaries were received; 7 did not take such cases, the 33 which did returned 347 cases. From 55 refuges the number of cases returned was 745; total for three years, 1092.

Some of the details are as follows:—8 cases between 6 and 8 years of age; 18 between 9 and 11 years; 11 cases of 12 years; 14 cases of 13 years; 121 cases of 14 years; and 301 cases of 15 years.

In one town the Chief Constable reports that hardly a child over 14 years has not fallen. From another, that children under 14 absolutely solicit in considerable numbers. In another, lads marked with badges solicit. On inquiring why prosecutions are so few, the reply comes from all quarters that so often the culprit is the father, step-father, uncle, or brother of the victim. In a covering letter, Mr. Cree writes that, besides the numbers already quoted, fully 1000 more cases were known, but the parents would not allow the rescue workers to deal with them.

He says convictions are *very* few, as relations are often the culprits, and prosecutions must be taken in hand within six months after the commission of the crime; and, when there is danger of an infant being born, the child is restrained by threats from saying anything until its state is manifest.

Also young children are subject to cross-examination by lawyers, and he states a case of a child of 10 being cross-examined for a full hour, but the evidence could not be shaken, and the case was sent to the Assizes.

From the Society for the Prevention of Cruelty

to Children came the statistics for last year—838 cases, 146 prosecuted, 46 being dismissed.

Of collected cases there are 20, 18 of these being under 16, one being only 3 and another 5 years of age. In two the fathers were the culprits, and in one the brother was suspected. In six of these cases nothing was done, either because parents would not prosecute, or for want of sufficient evidence. Two of these cases were very bad. One, a girl, went to a gardener's for fruit at midday on Sunday, did not return home until 6.30; then went out, presumably to chapel. Nothing more was seen of her until her body was taken from the river on the following Tuesday morning. On examination, the child was found to have been violated. The gardener was severely censured at the inquest, and an open verdict given.

The other was of a child of 12, who was outraged while her mother was lying dead. The child accused her father of the crime, but, as it could not be proved, he was let off.

Out of 11 cases which were investigated, 3 were discharged, 1 because there was, as the Judge said, "No corroboration," and 1 "not proven." Of the 6 convicted, 1 was let off with a fine, and the others received sentences varying from six months to ten years.

Of the two cases over 16, one was a girl of 17

mentally deficient, and the culprits (several youths, one of whom confessed to the wrong-doing) were all discharged by the magistrates. The other, also a girl of 17, was seized from behind, a drugged handkerchief stuffed into her mouth, and she was dragged into the bracken off the high road across a Surrey heath. There she was outraged, and when she recognised her assailant, he tried to pour poison down her throat, fortunately without much success. Chiefly because of the attempt to poison he got seven years. I think it should have been for life.

If such is the condition of things as they are known, what number of cases are there unknown? If there are 327 cases *reported* during a year, how very many hundreds are there unreported? Yet men who are supposed to protect the weak take every advantage of that weakness. Governments come and go, yet this terrible evil remains unchecked. Why have not these cases been put in the same category as murder? Do our law-makers consider it worse to kill the body than to outrage its honour and sully its soul?

It is useless to try, as some may do, to blame foreigners; only one culprit among all the reported cases for 1907 was an alien.

These men, who defile women and violate their own offspring, are British. They have the power of helping to make the laws which we women must obey, and, judging from these statistics, make them as easy as possible for the indulgence of their own lusts.

If this is not so, why must cases be instituted within six months of the offence? Why must a child, whose whole moral and physical nature has been so recently outraged, be subjected to cross-examination by a lawyer (a man) upon so delicate a matter?

And, lastly, how is it possible to expect corroborative evidence in the majority of such cases?

If such a state of things is the result of the absolute political power of men, the sooner women have votes the better it will be for the nation, and the sooner will its moral and physical condition be improved.

INADEQUATE PROTECTION TO GIRLS

" A sinister chapter to which too little attention has hitherto been paid is the failure of our legislatures and courts to afford to young girls protection from seduction, assault, and enslavement in infamous houses. The difficulty involved in obtaining the conviction of malefactors is known only to the few faithful souls who have attempted to obtain due punishment of these grave offences. Mothers in any community are more deeply stirred by these offences than by any others, but judges and juries vary beyond belief in their treatment of criminals guilty of crimes against girls.

" In one western State a woman worked fourteen years to obtain the enactment of a workable statute to punish crimes against female minors. At last such a law was passed and vigorously enforced. Fourteen criminals were sent to the penitentiary. Then a young lawyer offered his services to one of the criminals, to free him by showing that the law was unconstitutional because the title should have read '*to define and* punish crimes against female minors' whereas in fact the two words '*define and*' were missing from the title, though the necessary definition was contained in the body of the statute. Upon this frivolous ground the Supreme court of the State held the statute invalid, and nine of the fourteen criminals were forthwith freed. The others were too poor or too ignorant to obtain counsel, and they remained in the penitentiary."[1]

EXAMPLES OF LAWMAKING IN NEW YORK STATE

The maximum punishment that can be given to a "cadet," or man Section 1566 of the penal code of New York State, which is conspicu-

[1] *Woman Suffrage: its Relation to Working Women and Children*, by Florence Kelley, published by the National American Woman Suffrage Association.

who lives upon the earnings of prostitutes, in New York State is six months in the workhouse. The statute makes this offence a misdemeanour. ously placed in the surface cars fixes one year's imprisonment and $500 fine as the maximum penalty for stealing or giving away a transfer ticket worth five cents.

The offence of "procuring" is graver, and is punishable with the same degree of severity as is the offence of spitting on the floors of cars and public buildings.

APPENDIX D

PROTECTION OF WIDOWED MOTHERS

The possibilities of protection extended by the state to mothers with children who are dependent on them, not only for care but for a livelihood, are indicated by the systems of industrial insurance or compensation now in force in almost every civilised country except this one. Every European country, at the present time, compensates the widows of workmen who have been killed in industry. In England the widow receives a sum of money, while in most other countries she receives a pension equal to a part of her husband's earnings. This continues until she remarries, and serves to protect the orphans. In Germany the orphans are thus provided for until their fourteenth year,—the age at which they are allowed to begin earning.

One of the chief aims of the women of Australia, lately organised into a political association in order to concentrate effectively upon social legislation, is to bring about a higher degree of economic security for women who have children to support.

The idea that mothers, who provide citizens for the state, are as fully entitled to state support or pensions during the time when the children need their care as are soldiers, who fight for the state, is gradually making its way as a part of the new ideal.

The subject of industrial compensation may be found in *Workingmen's Insurance*, by William Franklin Willoughby, which is now under revision and is to be published by the Russell Sage Foundation. Of Australian methods Miss Alice Henry, Hull House, Chicago, writes that the united experience of all workers there supports the plan of the maternal subsidy. Its abuse may be readily prevented by careful administration. Though not yet universal, the practice of enabling deserving widows or deserted mothers to keep the home together is spreading in all the States. South Australia gives rations for children if more than one in a family. New South Wales, Western Australia, and Victoria board the children with their mothers to the age of twelve. See *Report* Interstate Conference of Workers among Dependent Children, and *Reports*, State Children's Department, Adelaide, Australia; also *State Children in Australia* by Miss Spence.

APPENDIX E

MINIMUM WAGE BOARDS

"The minimum wage boards were established . . . in response to an anti-sweating agitation. . . . The social sanction of the minimum wage determinations rests upon the common interest of society in maintaining among all classes of people a standard of living comporting with the general wealth and civilisation of the community, and guaranteeing healthy social progress. . . . Minimum wage boards . . . are composed of not less than four nor more than ten members representing equally the employers and employees in the trade under their jurisdiction with a chairman elected by the other members but who is not one of the original members of the board. A separate board is formed for each trade."

[*Bulletin of the Bureau of Labour*, vol. x., 1905, pp. 61, 62, Washington.]

" Equal pay for equal work has been partially recognised for the first time in Australia under private enterprise by a recent 'determination' of

Appendices

the Drapery Trade Wages Board. It is already in force in the Federal Public Service, in the Junior Grade of the State Education Department, and now a beginning has been made in private enterprise."

[Vida Goldstein in *Jus Suffragii*, organ of the International Woman Suffrage Alliance, January 15, 1910. Edited by M. G. Kramers, 92 Kruiskade, Rotterdam.]

APPENDIX F

THE LIQUOR TRAFFIC AND ITS ATTITUDE TOWARD WOMAN SUFFRAGE

The National American Woman Suffrage Association prints a leaflet reproducing what it calls a "secret circular" which was distributed by an association of brewers and wholesale liquor dealers in a western State at the time of a campaign to introduce a woman suffrage amendment into the State constitution. This circular came into the possession of the daily press and may be found in newspaper files. It is stated that its authenticity has never been denied. Part of its text runs as follows:

"It will take 50,000 votes to defeat woman suffrage; there are 2000 retailers in ———. That means that every retailer must bring in 25 votes on election day...

" We enclose 25 ballot tickets showing how to vote; we also enclose a postal card addressed to this association. If you will personally take 25 friendly voters to the polls on election day and give each one a ticket showing how to vote, please mail the postal card back to us at once. You need not sign the card. Every card has a number, and we will know who sent it in. Let us all pull together and let us all work. Let us each get 25 votes."

INDEX

A

Abolitionist Congress in Geneva, 77
" " " " resolutions of, 77-79
Accidental infection in syphilis, 31, 38-39
Acquired Syphilis, 10
Age of consent, U. S. laws concerning, 116-121
Ages when girls are ruined, 87-88
Alcoholism in syphilis, 15, 25-27
Antibodies, 10
Anti-serum treatment, gonorrhœa, 48

B

Blindness, in gonorrhœa, 46, 51
Breeding-place of the venereal diseases, 34
Brussels Conference, first, 81
" " resolutions, 83
" " second, 81, 83-89
" " resolutions, 89-90
Butler, Mrs. Josephine E., 69

C

Cancer and syphilis, 24
Chancroid, 52
Clandestine prostitution, 98, 99
Colles, phenomenon named after, 19
Congenital syphilis, 16-17
Constitutional forms of gonorrhœa, 46
Contagious Diseases Acts, The, 68
Continental System of Regulation of Vice, The, 66

Control of prostitution, 59–103
Course of gonorrhœa, 43
Crime and syphilis, 27–29
Crusade of women under Mrs. Butler, 71

D

Dangers of regulation, 93–103
Diplococcus gonorrhœæ, 40
Donné, 5
Double standard of morals, The, 60–62

E

Enfranchisement of women needed, 158–159, 164–166
Extent of prostitution, 152–154

G

Girls, trade in, 108–109
Gonococcus gonorrhœæ, 40
Gonorrhœa, 40
" and syphilis, 51, 52
" course of, 43
" history of, 41–43
" mortality from, in prostitutes, 50
" organism of, 40
Great Britain, regulation in, 67–75
Gummata, 16

H

Hard chancre, 12
Heredity, syphilis, 18
History, white slave trade, 104–105
Hours of work, 163

I

Immunity, gonorrhœa, 48
" syphilis, 20

Index

Incubation period { chancroid, 52; gonorrhœa, 43; syphilis, 11
Infantilism, 17
Initial sore of syphilis, 12
International Federation against vice, formation of, 77

L

Laws covering age of consent in U. S., 116–121
" share of, in white slave trade, 107–108
Legislation, efforts to amend, 109–110, 171 ff
Liquor traffic and woman suffrage, 186-187

M

Martineau, Harriet, warnings by, 68
Mediate contagion, 98
Metchnikoff, Élie, 5
Minimum wage boards, 185-186
Modes of transmission, gonorrhœa, 47-48
"   "   syphilis, 37-39
Moral standard, double, the, 60–62
Morals police. 64
Morbidity of gonorrhœa, 49
"   " syphilis, 29, 31
Mortality from gonorrhœa in prostitutes, 50
Mucous patch, syphilis, 13

N

National Consumers' League, inquiry into wages, 162–163
National Vigilance Leagues, 110–111
Need of knowledge, 133–136
Neisser, experimental work of, 9
"   micrococcus of, 40
"   serum diagnosis of, 9–10
Nervous system and syphilis, 22–24
Numbers of young men infected, 154-155

O

One-child sterility, 45

198   Index

P

Para-syphilitic diseases, 23
Pasteur Institute, 8
Persevering prostitutes, numbers of, 86
Poverty and prostitution, 156
Prevalence of gonorrhœa, 49
 " " syphilis, 29
Prevention of venereal diseases, 129–130
 " " " " (individual),138
 " " " " " childhood, 140–141
 " " " " " youth, 141–142
 " " " " " marriage, 143–145
 " " " " " accidental, 146–149
 " " " " (social) childhood, 160
 " " " " " girlhood, 162
 " " " " " motherhood, 160, 188–9
Primary lesion, syphilis, 12
 " stage " 12
 " " length of, 12
 " infection in gonorrhœa, 43
Profeta, phenomenon named for, 20
Progress of crusade against venereal disease, 74–75
Prostitutes, mortality of, gonorrhœa, 50
Prostitution, 34–36
 " of minor girls, 86
 " attempts at legislation in U. S., 171
Protest of women against regulated vice, 71
Puberty and syphilis, 17

R

Race suicide, the true, 52
Reasons for prostitution, 155–156
Regulation of prostitution, 59; efforts to secure legislation in
 U. S., 171
Regulationists in Medical Congress, 1873, 76
Report on Criminal Assault, 176 ff
Resolutions, first Brussels Conference, 83
 " second " " 89–90

Index

S

Sanitary inefficiency of regulation, 96–99
Schaudinn, discovery, of, 5–6
    "   organism of, 5
Second stage of gonorrhœa, 44–45
   "   "   " syphilis, 13–14
Select Committee, House of Commons, 75
   "   "   "   " Lords on white slave trade, 75
Share of laws, in white slave trade, 107–108
Social legislation needed, 163
Societies, Sanitary and Moral Prophylaxis, 90–91
Soft chancre, 52–53
Source and spread of syphilis, 32
Spirilla refringens, 6
Spirochæte balanitis, 7
    "   pallida, 5
    "   "   destroyed by heat, 7
    "   "   demonstrated in tissues, 8
Stages of gonorrhœa, 44–45
   "   " syphilis, primary, 11
   "   "   "   secondary, 13
   "   "   "   tertiary, 14
Statistics of gonorrhœa, 49–52
   "   " syphilis, 29–31
Sterility of gonorrhœa, 45–50
Struggle against Contagious Diseases Acts, 73–74
Supreme Court decision, 115
Syphilis, 3,
    "   acquired, 10
    "   and carcinoma, 24
    "   and crime, 27–29
    "   cause of, 4–5
    "   alcoholism in, 15, 25–27
    "   congenital, 10, 16–17
    "   course of, 10–11
    "   history of, 4
    "   mucous patches of, 13
    "   and the nervous system, 22–24

Syphilis, organism of, 5
" prevalence of, 29
" rash of, 13
" source of, 32
" stages of, 11-14
" statistics of, 29-31
" and tuberculosis, 24-25
" and gonorrhœa, 51, 52

T

Tertiary syphilis, 14
Third stage, gonorrhœa, 46
Three stages, gonorrhœa, 43
Tolerated houses, 65-67
Treponema pallidum, 7
Tuberculosis and syphilis, 24-25

V

Venereal sore, 52-53

W

White slave trade, Europe, 103-104
"   "   "   United States, 110-115
Widowed mothers, protection of, 185, 188-189

Y

Young men infected, numbers of, 154-155

Z

Zeissl, 22

"Status of the Nurse in the Working World"

Lavinia Dock's last address to a nurses' convention, in 1913 (<u>American Journal of Nursing</u> 13 [September 1913]: 971-975), urged the members of the American Nurses Association once more to reach out beyond their own working world. In asking understanding and sympathy for the labor movement, Dock spoke with authority. She herself had not only organized women workers on the Lower East Side but had searched the foreign language sources for Josephine Goldmark's <u>Fatigue and Efficiency</u>, a study of the effects of long working hours which stands as one of the landmarks of Progressive social research.

Dock's plea for support of other hospital workers' efforts to limit hours, and her suggestion that underpaid nurses might have a bond with underpaid "toilers" of the working class, would win more serious attention today than it did then. Nurses were uncertain of their status and middle-class opinion generally still hostile to unions and their largely immigrant membership.

STATUS OF THE NURSE IN THE WORKING WORLD

By LAVINIA L. DOCK, R.N.

I HAVE taken the liberty of altering two words in the title of my paper, so as to call it "The Relation of the Nurse to the Working World," for in considering the "status" of the nurse I did not feel clear what there was to say upon it, as her status in the world of work is assuredly one of unceasing change, growth, development. But as to her relative position to other workers in the world of work, it seems to me there is something for us all to study with some seriousness.

That the nurse is a worker no one can deny. However high professionally she may build her career, however distinguished and noble she may make it (and we all feel, thankfully, that the nature of our work sets no limits in these directions), she is still closely related to the world of workers whom we may call toilers. In this we may, if we will, see her most shining merit, for all those who think are now acknowledging that the labor of the world is the supreme service, and those who labor are the only real benefactors of society.

But there are still many who do not think, and they still need to be taught to see, the dignity, value, and essential nobility of work—the indispensable work which makes it possible for a civilization to arise—and to learn that parasitic idleness is the deepest disgrace of a modern human being. To help impress this lesson is an incidental part of our duty, imposed upon us involuntarily by our relation to the world of work. To teach it we need to know something more than many of us now know about that surrounding world. Krapotkin says that every specialist or expert ought to know enough of the work of other specialists or experts to understand and sympathize with what they have to do. And this is true for us. A vast field of human work and striving with which we are closely, though unknowingly, related, is the field of trades unionism. I remember well when my own ignorance of what the labor movement was and what it meant to humanity was profound and illimitable. I hope no other nurse is so uninformed, but I fear there are some who may be so. Life in the Settlement gave me the opportunity to learn what the labor movement was, with its yearning aspirations for a higher life and its boundless heroism and self-sacrifice, and left me without a doubt that it was within that movement Jesus of Nazareth taught two thousand years ago. Because we have not understood it, we and our professional brothers, the doctors, have fallen into a way of assuming a tone of superiority and aloofness which are funny examples of little human pride. Do let us learn to see that the trade unions are for workers the same that our organizations are for us—bonds of brotherhood and protection, designed for mutual aid, conference, stimulation and uplift. Their faults are like ours and the doctors'—faults of imperfect human nature which is going to school for the lessons of coöperative effort. We may have been excused for not knowing this movement so long as it was directly confined to men, but now that women and young girls down to fifteen years of age are in industry by the millions, and are also forming their protective and upreaching organizations, we are able to see that this movement is just another variant of our own.

The question then comes home, What is our relation to this world of work? I think the answer is: We are morally and honorably bound to do nothing that crushes it down and makes its struggle harder, and we should be glad and thankful to do everything we can to help it upward and onward.

The immediate demands of this world of work lie along three lines: Education, hours of work, wages.

As to education I think we do keenly realize and thoroughly understand our obligations to our less fortunate sisters. Our own sense of the needs of our own profession makes us insist on honest and sufficient educational standards, and in this we are helping all workers even though we are unconscious of doing so, for so close is our relation that every minimum standard we can fix and assure, helps to bring up standards for other groups and makes it easier for others to demand and to attain a fitting preparation.

As to hours of work we are not quite so clear-headed. We have not known enough history and so we have not understood what this vast immense world movement of labor for a shorter working day has been, and what its significance. Eager to throw ourselves into the crises of our own tasks, which are indescribably dramatic because they hinge always on the acutest questions of life and death, we have resented any interference with hours of work and have echoed the sentiment too often skilfully suggested by hospital directors personally nterested, that a "profession" must not become tainted with "trades unionism" and that legal ordering of working hours would savor of trades unionism and destroy professional ethics. All solemn pharisaism! And hospital directors know it is. And because our work is fascinating in the extreme, they have used us to help crush back the rightful demand of those co-workers whose work is purely laborious and devoid in itself of any dramatic or intellectual joy; those who deal only with dishes, mops, machines and drudgery. I am sorry to think how often, for instance, the great need for shorter hours of the workers in all kinds of hospital institutions in Massachusetts has been denied in the legislature with the help of nurses and doctors, who have appeared before it to declare that their professional honor would be injured if the law fixed hours of work. So because of their sensitive pride, other classes of toilers have been deprived of the protection that they needed. If you would clearly understand what overstrain is in the world of work read Josephine Goldmark's monumental book *Efficiency, Fatigue*. To the fact that I was privileged to collect some of this material for her, I owe all such knowledge as I have myself of the difference between work and overwork—the one, blessed, healthful, inspiring, even if the labor involved is of the humblest order—as it often must be—the other crushing, saddening, or brutalizing, destroying all joy in work, taking the light out of the day.

The whole long history of the labor movement shows the effort to so adjust the burden of toil that the worker may feel joy in his work. The struggle for the shorter working day is the struggle to live —to be a human being—to have a soul. It is this struggle we must learn to comprehend, for we have a relation to it that we do not now understand and there is a claim upon us which we are not fulfilling when we oppose legislation to limit the hours of work in hospitals.

As to wages, our conscience is again clear. We know that we must not undersell, that this is treachery to fellow workers, and helps to drag down even remote classes of such. Be it frankly admitted that this is a fundamental principle of unionism, and a most necessary and indispensable one, so long as we have our present social system. The material basis of life is the foundation on which we stand to build up the higher things, and if this basis is not secure, we all go down together. To the labor movement we owe examples of heroism and loyalty in holding this principle that we, a fortunate and on the whole privileged set of workers, have never yet been called on to imitate.

Society is not benefited by the presence of a poorly paid working class, nor by the ministrations of underpaid nurses, for the underpaid worker is liable at any moment to become a dependent, even a public charge, while from the standpoint of public health no class that is habitually overworked and underpaid ever shows a good grade of general healthfulness. Underpaid and underfed are synonymous terms, and we may therefore find a class of workers such as the cottage nurses of England who, presumably helping individuals in other classes to recover from illness, are by the conditions of this service being pressed downward into ill health and poverty. An example such as this proves that there are other and better ways, through an intelligent coöperation, of doing every kind of needed work without destroying the health and happiness of the worker. Our duty is undoubtedly to support every movement for an adequate-living wage for all workers, and, in this connection, I must allude to a recent newspaper controversy in a New York paper over the comparative salaries of nurses and teachers. Now teachers are notoriously grossly underpaid and it seemed clear to me that nurses, writing on this question to the papers, did not grasp the correct point. Instead of dwelling on the greater danger and uncertainty of a nurse's work, they should have insisted on the wretched inadequacy of the average teacher's wage, and have shown that, so far from nurses being paid too much, teachers are not paid enough.

You will hardly expect me to open my mouth without speaking of suffrage, and I do want to say most seriously that, in the world of work, the three needs of workers—education, shorter hours and a living wage —are terribly precarious, terribly uncertain, unstable and insecure unless protected well and firmly by legislation which is steadily and uniformly enforced by proper inspection and suitable penalties. And I should like to ask you to answer candidly this question. How likely is it that workers can secure such legislation and enforcement without the ballot? They are then a negligible quantity in the eyes of law-makers, and find a powerful body of employers armed with political power opposed to them. For the sake of the working woman, whose foothold is less secure than ours, no nurse should be opposed to enfranchisement for women. To climb up ourselves and push a weaker person down is what none of us would do by a physical act, and shall we do it by an attitude of mind? We have been privileged in our legislative success even without the vote, because every man has some grateful memory of a nurse, but we might have done even better had we had political power, and without it, can we feel sure of the future of our educational standards? The nurse of Great Britain, Germany, Holland, are badly oppressed and handicapped by their disfranchised state. How different is their status in the Scandinavian countries, Australia and New Zealand!

To close, it seems to me that our status in the working world will always be decided by the attitude that we take toward the needs and problems of the working world. If we are exclusive and shut our minds to all except "professional" subjects, we shall become one-sided specialists and in time lose our usefulness as did the French nuns in hospital work. If we acknowledge our relation to the working world, and fulfill the obligation that this relation brings, we shall live and become ever more useful and respected.

"Foreign Department"

To Lavinia Dock, the causes in which she enlisted were connected parts of an exhilarating lifetime effort for the one great cause of peace and justice. Women's suffrage took precedence in the strenuous final years of that campaign; it is our loss that she left no account of demonstrating and suffering imprisonment with other members of the National Woman's Party, the movement's militant left wing. But even then other parts of the larger crusade were not forgotten. One brief remark opposing the tactic of burning President Woodrow Wilson in effigy, "not for any personal feelings for Wilson but because it approaches so terribly to lynching," incidentally revealed her concern for the oppression of Negro Americans.

And always in the background as the suffrage struggle moved toward victory was the lengthening shadow of war. In 1916, preparing her monthly copy for the <u>American Journal of Nursing</u>'s Foreign Department--it was the Department's seventeenth year--she tried to explain the pacifist position opposing "preparedness" for which she, Lillian Wald, and others had been widely denounced. Once the United States became a combatant they refused to succumb to wartime propaganda and hatred of "the Hun." Lavinia Dock's final column for the Foreign Department, in March 1923, was a plea for help for German nurses, caught with their defeated nation in the trauma of runaway inflation. (<u>AJN</u> 17 [October 1916]: 58-59; 23 [December 1922, March 1923]: 209, 493.)

FOREIGN DEPARTMENT

IN CHARGE OF

LAVINIA L. DOCK, R.N.

LETTERS FROM DENMARK

Since the time of the San Francisco meetings no word had been received from Denmark in regard to the International Council of Nurses, until a few days ago. This was accounted for by us as a by-product of the world-war—of course an accidental, unintentional by-product, and this proves correct. A Danish nurse, arriving in New York recently brought letters from Mrs. Henny Tscherning, president of the International Council, including copies of those written a year ago and never received. Several from this side must also have been lost. Mrs. Tscherning, like the rest of us, feels dubious as to the near possibility of a truly successful meeting of the International Council of Nurses in a European country. For my part, as secretary of the Council, it seems clear that we must prepare to push our next meeting date a little further on than 1918, as the continuance of war is making it too close to give us time to prepare for a date only a little more than a year off. And, as it was our country's turn to hold a Congress and only a business meeting was possible at San Francisco, it might be better for us to make another attempt, when the time does come, to hold the next meeting here.

In this connection I would like to emphasize afresh and with a little more explanation the point of view of some of us on this side—Miss Wald and the whole Settlement group, and others, as to preparedness for war—why we oppose and resist it. It has not needed the tragic and terrible example of Europe to inspire our sentiments, neither are we lacking in profound sympathy for the nations so fearfully afflicted.

War is an integral part of the competitive system. It is the flower and fruit of competition. In war, such as rages in Europe, we see only the inevitable, acute stage of industrial and commercial warfare which is present with us all, in more or less sub-acute stages, wherever cut-throat competition is the accepted policy.

We believe that coöperation is the law of life and growth; competition, of destruction and death. War is avoidable through men's actions. It does not come by natural agencies like flood or lightning or cyclone, it is not even like a contagious disease, which is indeed spread by man's ignorance or carelessness, but without plan or purpose on his part. War arises from man's actions toward his brother man, his words to him, his feelings toward him. In proportion as he practices justice and regard for others, war is preventable. As he indulges jealousy and hatred, war is inevitable.

And we regard preparedness for war as a hot house and cultivator for jealousy, suspicion and hatred. Energies devoted to preparation for war are energies taken away from the saving, wholesome, living forces of international friendship and coöperation. No one can at one and the same time work for competition and for coöperation. Each must choose one or the other,

The nations plunged over the abyss at the end of their competitive race could at last, when the crisis came, do no other than they have done. But now if ever is the time for ours and all neutral countries to recognize the peril of national shortsightedness and to assert more strongly than before the saving power of the International Idea—the world our one common country, international association and organization for world law the only hope for the future.

FOREIGN DEPARTMENT

Lavinia L. Dock, R.N., Department Editor

AS Christmas draws near, every friend of mankind must ask himself how near he comes to fulfilling the words: "Love your enemies." Many, many professing Christians asked this question during the war, became angry and replied that it was a holy duty to hate Germans. I hope that nurses do not share this view, for German nurses are in serious distress because of the generally terrible and disastrous effect of the peace, so-called, for it is really not yet peace but cruel financial war still going on that keeps the middle classes especially, in Europe, in poverty and distress.

I do not know what we can do to help our German sisters. The problem is too vast and complicated for individual help to seem anything but a drop in the bucket. They have not asked us for help, nor uttered a complaint. This groping tentative suggestion is my own, and yet I hardly know what to suggest, except that, if any group or alumnae society wishes to send any gift to Sister Agnes Karll, at the German Nurses' Association, Regensburger Str. 28 IV., Berlin W. 50, I know that she will apply it to help some one in special need.

Whoever was to blame for the war, the nurses certainly were not, and now that Germany has overthrown her imperialism and is struggling along the paths of democracy, with plain men and women doing wonderful work in altering school text books to cast out all teaching of nationalistic egoism, she deserves the sympathy and help of others with the same ideals.

If we must hate anything, let it be the tendency, the emotionality, of economic imperialism wherever found,—but not any other human being.

L. L. Dock.

FOREIGN DEPARTMENT

Lavinia L. Dock, Department Editor

SISTER Agnes Karll writes with touching appreciation and responsiveness in regard to gifts of money which are reaching her from American nurses. She is able to make every dollar go to its utmost in relieving pathetic cases of illness, breakdown, or destitution from unemployment among the older Sisters.

The newspapers make it perfectly plain that the middle classes of Germany are undergoing severe hardships and as it is to that class that nurses, medical men, teachers, etc., belong, we may realize what it means to them when the cost of living doubles over night.

One would think that the world generally would feel some wish to help a country which has thrown off its imperialistic militarism; which has enfranchised women and given them seats in Parliament; which has been taking "hate teachings" out of the school books; which has become a republic with a sincere, upright working-class President; which is now offering only "passive resistance," moral force, to physical force.

But instead, sadly enough, the opposite seems to be the case and it often seems as if the young, struggling Republic were detested more than the autocratic Empire, and as if other countries were more determined now, to kill out a dawning democracy than ever they were of old to get rid of Empires and Emperors. Meanwhile the nurses are thankful for the help we can send them.

(In the December *Journal* it was requested that contributions for German nurses should be sent to Sister Agnes Karll. Sister Agnes has been recently called to her mother who is ill, in a country place, so contributions may be addressed, instead, to Berufsorganisation, Regensburger Str. 28 IV, Berlin, W. 50, Germany.)

"Letters to the Editor"

This exchange of Letters to the Editor (American Journal of Nursing 24 [May, July 1924]: 665-666, 834) reflects, in the single area of the nursing profession, the schism that divided and weakened feminists in the 1920s almost from the moment of the suffrage victory.

Lavinia Dock is defending a leaflet she had widely distributed in December 1923 calling upon nurses to support the Equal Rights Amendment, first introduced that year by the National Woman's Party. Fifty years later, in the 1970s, the ERA would be passed by Congress and come close to ratification; in the 1920s its supporters were only a small minority. Most feminists and reformers in general opposed the amendment on the ground that it would invalidate the social legislation protecting women for which they had fought hard during the Progressive years.

EQUAL RIGHTS

DEAR EDITOR: In view of the fact that a printed letter with the name of a well known nurse at the end of it has been sent to many nurses to call their attention to the so-called "equal rights" amendment to the Federal Constitution, the undersigned desire to point out certain matters in connection with the proposed legislation which should be of interest to nurses. The amendment referred to, which is sponsored by the National Women's Party, reads:

"Section 1. Men and women shall have equal rights throughout the United States and every place subject to its jurisdiction.

"Section 2. Congress shall have power to enforce this article by appropriate legislation."

Nurses should know that while the amendment has a plausible sound, and at the first glance might seem well worth supporting, it could not do what it purports to do; and moreover, that Congress or the states already have the power to do what the amendment is supposed to bring about. Most women as a general principle want equal rights, but certainly the thoughtful ones will see that an act which would invalidate beneficial labor laws for women, and laws providing pensions for widowed or dependent mothers, or age-of-consent laws for girls, and other laws applying to women and not to men, cannot mean an improvement for women in general. Such thoughtful ones should advocate specific laws to correct specific discrimination against women, and would oppose blanket legislation which not only is unnecessary, but would involve endless litigation, to determine the meaning of the terms "rights" and "equal rights." It has been demonstrated that the method of specific laws to correct specific discrimination against women is feasible, for women have succeeded in the three years since the federal suffrage amendment was ratified in removing sixty-eight such discriminations in the laws of twenty-eight states. Nurses should know that opposed to the National Women's Party Amendment are:

National League of Women Voters
National Consumers League

National Women's Trade Union League
American Federation of Labor
American Federation of Teachers
National Council of Jewish Women
National Council of Catholic Women
General Federation of Women's Clubs
American Home Economics Association
National Council of Women
Girls' Friendly Society in America
Young Women's Christian Association
United Textile Workers
Republican National Committee
Democratic National Committee
American Association of University Women.

Is this not a good company in which to be? The organizations opposing the blanket amendment are not opposing equal rights for men and women, as some of them are definitely working for legislation for this purpose in the states. The opposition is directed toward the blanket method of legislation because of the uncertainty as to the legal situation, if such an amendment to the Constitution should be passed. Few people are in a position to know more about the harm the proposed amendment would do than the Chief of the Children's Bureau, and the Chief of the Women's Bureau. Both Miss Grace Abbott and Miss Mary Anderson are strongly opposed to the amendment. Should not nurses ally themselves with the strong body of women who are working against the bill? This is the personal opinion of the undersigned and does not express that of the groups which they represent.

JULIA C. STIMSON,
Major, Supt., Army Nurse Corps.
J. BEATRICE BOWMAN,
Supt., Navy Nurse Corps.
LUCY MINNIGERODE,
Supt., U. S. Public Health Nursing Service.
MARY A. HICKEY,
Supt. of Nurses, U. S. Veterans' Bureau.

LETTERS TO THE EDITOR

The editors are not responsible for opinions expressed in this department. Letters should not exceed 250 words and should be accompanied by the name and address of the writer.

EQUAL RIGHTS

DEAR EDITOR: In the discussion of what an "Equal Rights" amendment to the United States Constitution may or may not do for the position of women it may be pointed out that the whole subject of mothers' or widows' pensions and maternity aid is coming to be differently regarded by workers and authorities in those social reforms. Such measures are now seen to be for the benefit of the race instead of merely aid to women. The Children's Bureau which used to use the term "Mothers' Pensions" now writes in a recent publication: "The earlier familiar title * * * Mothers' pensions * * * is becoming obsolete. * * * The emphasis is being placed on Home Care for Children." Judge Lindsey says: "I heartily favor the Equal Rights Amendment. * * * Special legislation is in fact not for women at all, but for children. Colorado makes no distinction as to parent." The Colorado law says: "A parent or other person" in its provision for dependent or neglected children,—we may soon, therefore, see widowed fathers receiving "maintenance for children," and why not? Fears for the Sheppard Towner Act under Equal Rights are already subsiding as it is clear that all babies born are not girls and that husbands are equally benefited by a reduced death rate of mothers in childbirth and a diminished infant mortality. Age-of-consent laws would certainly be more effective if applied to both boys and girls and here, too, as a matter of fact, we find examples where progressive states are now legally protecting the youth of both sexes against sex offenses. There is a glimpse of future possibilities here. Labor legislation presents the strongest case in opposition, because men don't want it for themselves. Yet this too is full of danger if applied only to women,—consider what the results will be if the legal exclusion of women from opportunities to work be extensively attained throughout all our states. They will be pushed back into the position they were in a hundred years ago, and it will not be easy to break through again if shut out by specific legislation. The wretched strain and struggle and overwork in our labor world are caused basically by poverty and it will not help that to make it harder for women to find self-support. A quite different treatment is indicated for the disease of poverty. Moreover we claim that the very reason women have been handicapped in competing with men is the inferior position which custom, the common law, and the canon law have heretofore given them. It has put them in the class with aliens. We must get them out of this. A good Labor Party, such as seems now to be on the way, should offer the best promise of dealing effectively with the conditions of labor in the future for men and women both. We might then arrive at: 1. Ample protection for boys and girls up to a given age (this protection has, so far, I fear, been hindered by the frequent linking of "Women and Children" together in attempts to legislate). 2. Equal conditions of protection for young workers of both sexes in industry. 3. Equal rights and opportunities for adult men and women without restriction or exclusion based on sex alone —such restriction or exclusion to be based only on physical fitness, or age, or the dangers of an occupation, or general hygiene applicable to human beings. Women would then be able to give men a lead—not just tag submissively after them in industry. Motherhood as we have pointed out is a race service and it is possible that fatherhood may also come to be so regarded. We are beginning to learn that sterility may be traced to an overworked father. We must come to see that all labor legislation should aim at health conservation. Now, health is not a sex privilege. We claim, too, that fundamental rights of citizens should be declared in our federal constitution, not left to the several states. State laws are too easily altered or overthrown by selfish elements and too difficult of improvement by reform elements.

Pennsylvania   LAVINIA L. DOCK.

"Lavinia L. Dock: Self-Portrait"

An inquiry from the American Journal of Nursing in 1932 caught the seventy-six-year-old Dock in a mellow mood and elicited this insightful and typically candid memoir.

(Copyright (c) 1977, American Journal of Nursing Company. Reproduced with permission from Nursing Outlook, Vol. 25, No. 1, January 1977, pages 22-26.)

In 1932, in response to a request from the American Journal of Nursing Company, Lavinia Dock provided what she calls in a covering letter the "little biographical sketch that I promised." Never published, it was stored in the Nursing Archive of Boston University's Mugar Memorial Library, along with other historical materials of the Journal Company. Identified by Mary Ann Garrigan, curator of the nursing archive and professor of nursing at Boston University, as a valuable historical document, it is published here for the first time. Written in longhand and addressed to a member of the American Journal of Nursing staff, it is reproduced exactly as Miss Dock wrote it, save for occasional modifications in punctuation where it was difficult to decipher exactly what Miss Dock had intended.

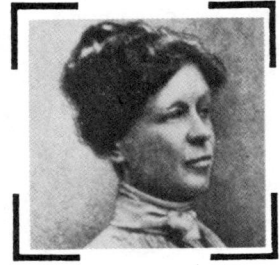

LAVINIA L. DOCK: Self-Portrait

July 6, 1932

Dear Mrs. Stevens,

The things going on in the world today make my history more than ever of no importance, but I know that Editors <u>must</u> get copy so I will try to help you out.

I was born in 1858 in Harrisburg where both my parents homes were and grandparents lived and where we have also lived off and on though while we were all little children we were for some years in the coal regions of Dauphin Co. where my father had posts.

Both my grandfathers were of German descent but born in this country—both good, upright, industrious citizens of the middle class. Both of them amassed a fair amount of property in land which was partly lost in the crash of 1873, kept us "landpoor" (paying taxes) for some years, then becoming valuable. Gave my sisters and self modest incomes (which are now disappearing in the crash of 1929-32). One of my grandfathers was a friend of Dorothea Dix and took an active part in helping her work for a State Hosp near Harrisburg. His name is on a tablet in the hospital.

The other was interested in various worthy but bourgeois doings such as founding a bank and sitting as "judge" in the rather informal court for municipal matters of those days.

Both the grandmothers were American born—one of English (unorthodox Quaker-Hicksite) folk, the other of French immigrants—supposedly Huguenot—to the Southern states. While there was nothing specially distinguished about any of them yet they all had some ideas of their own.

My parents were well taught for their day and their small town and were both of liberal views—my mother especially so. Father had some whimsical masculine prejudices but Mother was broad on all subjects and very tolerant and charitable toward persons.

They both went to church but we children were never made to go nor do I remember ever hearing religion talked of at home. We never heard the words "sin" or "wicked." I am certain that neither one believed in "hell" tho my mother believed in a future (happy) life.

We were taught that things were "honorable" or "dishonorable" or were "common" (meaning low or base). To use the word "lie" would have been utterly shocking. "Truthful" and "untruthful" were high lights among words. One of the most grievous offences was to say illnatured things about anyone. Father could, as I learned later, condemn and judge persons severely tho justly. I never heard my mother gossip or talk over other people's private affairs or characters. Either some excuse or good quality would be mentioned, or else silence.

In some ways I was a bright child, in others very dense and slow. I learned to read at an unusually early age and read all sorts of everything but had few definite thoughts—no quick wit —made no bright remarks. As we grew up we girls were educated in "nice" private schools where the teaching was oldfashioned and conventional. There I was very superficial, learning easily and quickly the things I liked (music-French-history) and utterly refusing any effort for what I disliked (grammar-arithmetic-dates-names of kings etc.). I had a facility for getting away with this. My teachers liked me but said I lacked application and was not "ambitious."

In my youth I showed none of the qualities needed for a good nurse. I was easily satisfied, happy-go-lucky, not exactly dreamy, but placid and good-humored generally, with a quick flash of temper sometimes which was soon over and forgotten. I was fond of outdoors—of the features of nature, the hills and the little streams, and of pets. I never cared for dolls nor had any—I was also forgetful—a bad fault.

Until well on in my teens I had never had occasion to think of illness—nor had the concept "hospital" come into my mind in any way. When I was 18, my mother died after a rather short illness, and I then showed (as she thought) some instinctive gift at making her comfortable, more than the others. But that experience did not turn my thoughts to nursing as it has done with many others. I remained unconscious and unthinking, but rather practical and steady in helping with [sic] my older sister, with the care of younger ones.

There were however two rather curious incidents that seem to show inherited memory. The first one: I think I was not more than eight or nine years old when I read in a Boston paper a news item about a nurse who had infected a finger, and about the treatment of it. A curious sense of knowing about it came as I read—it seemed familiar. But this feeling passed off and I gave it no thought. It has however always stayed in my memory as rather inexplicable.

The second: After my mother's death there was a serious business crash. Everyone was poor and my father had serious financial struggles. Nevertheless, it was unheard of then for girls of our class to earn their livings. There were of course a few exceptions. Teachers: they were born, we supposed. No matter how poor "nice" families were they scraped and pinched and would have been horrified at the thought of girls doing anything but live at home.

But one day my older sister said to me "If Father was ruined and we had to go out to work (that was the expression then) what would you do?"

Without a moment's hesitation and yet without ever before having had a thought of the kind, or of any kind I replied "I would go and work in a hospital." Having said that I never thought of it again nor do I know why I said it. It was not until some years later that I read the Century article containing the cut of Isabel Hampton. That really did give me a definite thought and led me to definite steps. I went to Bellevue in 1884.

You will not like to tell your inquirers that I was never a really good nurse yet that is the truth. I continued to be too easily satisfied—not keenly observant—hazy, rather than dreamy—not sufficiently vigilant—too optimistic—I continued to wish only to do the things I liked—my feelings for my patients were compassion, or commiseration, or sympathy, rather than a warm personal care.

I was not unconscious of my defects but never eradicated them. As I think now, they rested upon a physical basis. My thumbs and little fingers do not match;—my nose is the wrong shape;—one ear has distinctly a pointed tip and so on.

In hospital work I was better in the assisting than in the leading position. I never had jealousy or envy. These were sensations entirely unknown. I was, rather, enthusiastic in admiration and esteem for others. I have been called "an appreciator" and believe this was correct.

[Miss Palmer (Sophia) at one time (because we were in disagreement over various things) thought me jealous and trying to undermine her but in this she was wholly mistaken. Certain attitudes of hers in international affairs I did want her to alter. Otherwise I always admired her strong character and great ability. As for wanting to be Journal editor myself I would have run away without stopping, rather.]*

I was very faithful and diligent at the Johns Hopkins, and happy. At the Cook County I

---

*Brackets are Miss Dock's.

was really a failure. Let me say that, looking back I can confidently assert that my principles, aims, and endeavors were right and sound, but I showed no diplomatic skill in personal relations. I was not careful enough in avoiding trouble beforehand.

I have often been glad since then that my stay there was short or I might have missed my happy years at Henry Street, in writing History and helping international organizations. For my mind was a one-track one and in absorption over the immediate I lost sight of the horizon. It is odd that at that time an old friend—Miss Woodworth of Bellevue said to me: "What you should do now is to write"—I laughed at her, thought the idea comic.

My father died and I spent more than a year at home in order that my oldest sister could go away to prepare herself for what was to be her very important and really distinguished life work: i.e.—teaching plant biology and botany. She became eminent in horticulture, park development and town planning, civic work of all kinds and finally in state forestry, and was made a member of the State Forestry Commission—an unpaid post of importance which she held for many years. I think that, as the others were younger she might not have been able to take the university work had I not been at home and have always regarded that as one of the fortunate turns in events in my rather unplanned life.

I never began to think until I went to Henry Street, and lived with Miss Wald. I was then about 38 years old. But as I then began to reflect I saw that I had always had certain inarticulate instincts that were sound:—a strong sympathy with oppressed classes, a lively sense of justice and a keen love of what we mean by "freedom" and "liberty"— My first experiments in thinking showed me that I had no religious beliefs and that I felt no need of them.

In early life I had gone to church and Sunday school because the other girls did. For several years I had played the organ in a small church because of my love of music. I took for granted that I believed the doctrines I heard and to this day am fond of the hymns and have always been glad of hearing so much of the poetry legend and prophecy of the Bible (Episcopal Church). My first instinctive revolt was in the hospital when I saw an emergency birth. The flash went through my mind: "There is not a good God!" But I went no further then. Later in the Spanish American war, to which of course all liberals were intensely opposed I heard a clergyman— a most excellent and good sincere man defend our conquest of the Philippines and say: "They (the natives) have no business to resist us."

Instantly all regard for and belief in the Church as an institution fell out of my mind as a stone sinks in water, and never came back. Years before that the histories of the Civil War time and the defence of slavery made by the churches had deeply impressed my emotions but I did not then think it out. Now I one day recited to myself the Apostles Creed in order to see what I believed. I found that I only accepted the two last words "Life everlasting" but the life I believed in was what we see in nature and not the immortality of the individual.

Incidentally I may add that the idea of eternal life for individual persons is to me a terrible one and not at all to be wished for—Imagine meeting William Randolph Hearst and knowing that he was going to live forever!! No pain or sense of loss accompanied my disbelief. On the contrary as I saw more of the misery and cruelty of human beings and read more of the long ages and milleniums of slavery, cruelty and pain I would have felt horror of an omnipotent God who could preside over such suffering and now I feel confident that whatever the vast creative power is—it has no human feelings;—does not care or know. The presence of love and kindness in human beings (and also in animals) I interpret as being the effect wrought into living cells by sunlight or rays of light. This would be no more wonderful than the springtime in Nature.

A change came about in my feelings toward Jesus. So long as I thought that I believed he was a divinity I could feel none of the gratitude and devotion for him that the clergy told us we should feel. I often tried in vain to reach this emotion. It seemed to me that, if a deity had condemned the human race after creating it, 'twas no more than he should do, to save it. Very different were my sensations as I came to see him as a humble Jewish working man—one of the long line of such martyrs and prophets in the ages. Then, gratitude and reverence and love came fully without artificial stimulation.

All this became plain to me in my life on the East Side as there I met in person working men of exactly the type of Jesus—learned of their lifelong ideals for a better life for all humanity and saw their struggles and their persecution in the Labor Movement. Learning something of the historic labor movement and its significance for humanity I became a radical in my opinions—hopes, and beliefs. Alas I have to confess, not in my life, and this duality is a constant source of sadness. But I see no way possible for me to live as a radical. I appear to have duties to my sisters now that we are all old and growing feeble and it would offend my common sense (of which I have a good deal) to refuse the near duties for distant ones. Yet that is what the true revolutionaries do and it is what Jesus said should be done. I content myself with voting the socialist tickets. Socialists deplore violence and believe in the appeal to Reason. I firmly believe that only by some mode of communistic ownership and sharing of wealth can there be any hope of a social system, better than this crazy, mad one that we have when millions starve while boundless resources are available, and food is burned or thrown into the ocean to keep prices up.

The intellectual and idealistic Jews of international outlook and sympathies that I met seemed to me the highest type of civilized man. Their clear, noble thoughts and finely tempered minds always gave me the impression of being in the presence of a superior race and I do think that as instruments of thought and intellectual, moral, and spiritual penetration and perceptions no other minds quite equal theirs. Miss Wald's nature seemed to me to surpass any other that I knew. Like the sun, she radiated her beams on all without demands or exactions for a return.

While I came rather late to economic fields the woman movement [sic] had been more nearly born in me. I could not have been more than twelve when I read some of the earliest challenges thrown out by defiant women and these aroused a fellow feeling in my inner self. It was a great joy to do a little guerilla war in that cause and I believe that going to jail gave me a purer feeling of unalloyed content than I ever had in any of my other work where I always saw some imperfections to cause chagrin.

No sooner was that movement over than I found I must take the opposition to almost all my old friends because it became clear that the vote must only be the tool by which to gain complete legal equality the world over by getting rid of discriminatory laws of which many hundreds defied partial and local efforts. The vision of world womanhood still kept under by discriminations based on sex only, showed that the so called protective labor legislation—in which I once believed and which was right enough so long as women were disfranchised—was only a form of segregation, and under a fair pretense, was really only a method for keeping women classed with children.

I am quite certain that, under international charters of legal and economic equality with men—all those differences that do arise from sex would settle themselves just as physical differences between man and man settle themselves.

In the untrammeled power of workingwomen to unite with men in getting improvements for all labor and especially for children I see a great force now wasted or shackled. So I do not mind having lost some old friends on this issue for the thing is more important.

Shall I touch on the sentimental, or rather the unsentimental? Well we girls grew up freely with boys and young men—with no special incidents. When I was about seventeen I spent a week with some married friends who had staying with them a young Polish violinist—then quite famous—Adamowski.

I did not think of him as a handsome young man but did feel awed by the fact of his being a famous musician and I greatly enjoyed his sitting beside the piano humming and beating time while I played (quite nicely for I had a good touch).

One day I overheard him say to my hostess, in a casual, patronizing tone: "She would make a good wife." Something in his manner conveyed a sense of inferiority. I felt keen mortification—also a sense of alarm. In a flash I seemed to see my freedom gone, myself perhaps a household drudge, and no way out. I said to myself "I never will" and that impression stayed with me all my life.

I never felt attracted to the domestic hearth. Nor did I ever want children of my own. Yet I am fond of the little things and can't endure seeing them mistreated or misunderstood. As a little girl I had read Victor Hugo's Les Misérables and never forgot the picture of little Cosette carrying her heavy pails of water. I think too that perhaps Hugo's (no doubt sentimentalized) convict prepared my mind for the later more enlightened horror of our stupid, cruel, and barbarous prison system. As I grew older and saw the world it seemed to me dreadful to bring more children into the world while so many were neglected and abused. I still think so and firmly advocate "Birth Strikes" against war and birth control thro universal, dignified, professional instruction.

The only piece of work that I ever thought of myself was the Materia Medica. I had no advice, no consultation with anyone. It came into my own head and all by myself I wrote letters, without knowing how, to all the big men asking their permission to use their books. I am rather pleased with that, for you can see that, generally speaking, I did not originate, and rather needed some stimulus from other minds to start me on a track.

I had very kind replies—a most courteous, polished one from the Englishman Lauder Brunton and a sharp one from Dr. Wood of Phila. telling me not to Eviscerate his enormous book. I prepared it one year while Night Superintendent at Bellevue, writing it in the mornings and copying it at night. I showed it to no one, nor spoke of it until it was done. Sent it to Putnams with all my letters by messenger. The letters in some way were lost and they sent in bewilderment to look me up to ask what it was.

They were not willing to publish it at their own expense but, without a doubt or a qualm, in perfect certainty I told them I would pay for it. I borrowed the money from my father who was certain I was gambling on a gold brick, but within a year I began paying him back.

I thought of it because we then had to buy a number of expensive books. The Drs. gave large doses of deadly poisons and expected the nurses to watch the results and not allow any untoward effects. I tried therefore to gather every word on symptoms and signs—also, drugs were fluid and mostly given by mouth. Being very nasty we were expected to learn how to make them less so and I collected every recipe I could find or hear of. I have been told that, because the early editions were full of practical details on those two special points, many medical students bought the book. As times changed all that of course became also passé.

The little book had quite a run and at its highest point sold over 6,000 copies in a year.

The History I would never in the world have thought of by myself. It was entirely Miss Nuttings doing as it had been her dream. I think I never enjoyed anything more than working with her on that book. It was delightful from beginning to end and all the digging in public libraries, translating, researching and correcting was pure pleasure.

Because she was head of the JHH school, to do much of it herself was out of the question. Overburdened with many cares, she had no time for writing. She did however write two chapters and I have never found anyone who could pick them out. We never told anyone which ones they were but I will tell you now that she wrote the chapter on Early Nursing in Canada, and that on the Knightly nursing orders. Her style is more brilliant than mine and her vocabulary much more distinguished. However the whole book was gone over by Dr. Smith at the JHH who corrected everybody's English. Possibly for this reason the difference in style was less noticeable.

Miss Nutting also suggested the Short History but that never gave me the joy that the long one did. The last edition, which is much the best owes its finish and good balance to Miss Stewart as well as its attractive illustrations. She also wrote the Preface, and the final chapter, arranged all lists of recommended reading and made the various appendices.

I have written enough I think. I have tried to be truthful but perhaps have not told all the truth. Probably no one ever quite tells all they know about themselves.

If I could have three wishes for qualities in which I have always been deficient I would wish for:
    Keen observation and perception
    An excellent memory
    More affection for the individual person

                                Lavinia L. Dock

LAVINIA DOCK

SELECTED BIBLIOGRAPHY

Text-book of Materia Medica for Nurses. New York: G.P. Putnam's Sons, 1890.

"The American Pension Fund for Nurses." Trained Nurse and Hospital Review 8 (June 1892): 257-257.

"The Question of Nurses' Directories." Trained Nurse and Hospital Review 13 (October 1894): 171-174.

"The Editor's Letter-Box" [Pension fund letters]. Trained Nurse and Hospital Review 14 (June 1895): 347-350, and 15 (July 1895): 37.

"The Relation of Training Schools to Hospitals." Hospitals, Dispensaries and Nursing, John Shaw Billings and Henry M. Hurd, eds. Baltimore, 1894.

"The Non-Payment System as Established in the Illinois Training School." Society of Superintendents, Proceedings, January 1894.

"Directories for Nurses." Society of Superintendents, Proceedings, February 1895.

"A National Association for Nurses and Its Legal Organization." Society of Superintendents, Proceedings, 1896.

"Louise Darche, A Reformer in Nursing and in the Civil Service." Trained Nurse and Hospital Review 23 (October 1899): 195-201.

"What We May Expect from the Law." American Journal of Nursing 1 (October 1900): 8-12.

"The International Council of Nurses." AJN 1 (November 1900): 114-115.

Short Papers on Nursing Subjects. New York: M. Louise Longeway, 1900.

"The School-Nurse Experiment in New York." AJN 3 (November 1902): 108-110.

"Hospital Organization." National Hospital Record 6 (1903): 10-14.

"The Duty of This Society in Public Work." Society of Superintendents, Proceedings, 1903; AJN 4 (November 1903): 99-101.

"Is the Profession Becoming Overcrowded?" AJN 3 (April 1903): 513-515.

"An Experiment in Contagious Nursing." Charities 11 (July 4, 1903): 19-23.

"Spread of Visiting Nursing." Charities and the Commons 16 (April 7, 1906): 1-6.

"Central Directories and Sliding Scales." AJN 7 (October 1906).

"Some Urgent Social Claims." AJN 7 (1907): 895-905.

A History of Nursing [with Adelaide Nutting]. Volumes 1 and 2. New York: G.P. Putnam's Sons, 1907.

"Almshouse Nursing." AJN 8 (February 1908): 361-363.

"The Crusade for Almshouse Nursing." AJN 8 (April 1908): 520-523.

"The International Congress on Tuberculosis in Washington." AJN 9 (November 1908): 93-97.

"The London Meeting of the International Council and Congress of Nurses." AJN 10 (October 1909):

15-21.

"Recollections of Miss Hampton at the Johns Hopkins."
AJN 11 (October 1910).

Hygiene and Morality: A Manual for Nurses and Others, Giving an Outline of the Medical, Social, and Legal Aspects of the Venereal Diseases. New York: G.P. Putnam's Sons, 1910.

A History of Nursing. Volumes 3 and 4. New York: G.P. Putnam's Sons, 1912.

"The Isabel Hampton Robb Memorial Fund." The Johns Hopkins Nurses' Alumnae Magazine 11 (April 1912).

"The Status of the Nurse in the Working World." AJN 13 (September 1913): 971-975.

"Foreign Department." AJN 17 (October 1916): 58-59; 23 (December 1922, March 1923): 209, 493.

"Letters to the Editor" [Equal Rights Amendment]. AJN 24 (May, July 1924): 665-666, 834.

History of Red Cross Nursing [with others]. New York: The Macmillan Co., 1922.

"Our Debt to the Woman Movement." University of Pennsylvania Hospital Training School Alumnae Association, The Nurses' Quarterly 7 (September 1929).

A Short History of Nursing [with Isabel M. Stewart]. New York: G.P. Putnam's Sons, 1920, 1925, 1931, 1938.

"Lavinia L. Dock: Self-Portrait" [1932]. Nursing Outlook 25 (January 1977): 22-26.

"When We Wrote a History." The Johns Hopkins Nurses' Alumnae Magazine 49 (April 1950), 59-60.

Titles in This Series

1   Charlotte Aikens, editor. *Hospital Management.* Philadelphia, 1911.

2   American Society of Superintendents of Training Schools for Nurses. *Annual Conventions*, 1893–1919.

3   John Shaw Billings and Henry M. Hurd, editors. *Hospitals, Dispensaries and Nursing: Papers and Discussion in the International Congress of Charities, Correction and Philanthropy.* Baltimore, 1894.

4   Annie M. Brainard. *The Evolution of Public Health Nursing.* Philadelphia, 1922.

5   Marie Campbell. *Folks Do Get Born.* New York, 1946.

6   *Civil War Nursing:* Louisa May Alcott. *Hospital Sketches.* Boston, 1863. BOUND WITH *Memoir of Emily Elizabeth Parsons.* Boston, 1880.

7   Committee for the Study of Nursing Education. *Nursing and Nursing Education in the United States.* New York, 1923.

8   Committee on the Grading of Nursing Schools. *Nurses, Patients and Pocketbooks.* New York, 1928.

9   Mrs. Darce Craven. *A Guide to District Nurses.* London, 1889.

10   Dorothy Deming. *The Practical Nurse.* New York, 1947.

11   Katharine J. Densford & Millard S. Everett. *Ethics for Modern Nurses.* Philadelphia, 1946.

12   Katharine D. DeWitt. *Private Duty Nursing.* Philadelphia, 1917.

13   Janet James, editor. *A Lavinia Dock Reader.*